Sometimes They Forget

Finding Hope in the Alzheimer's Journey

RJ Thesman

DEDICATION

To my parents, Henry and Arlene Ediger,
who walked their journeys with grace and strength.

TABLE OF CONTENTS

ACKNOWLEDGMENTS

Every author has a group of people who help make the final draft exactly as the author intended. I feel blessed to add these people to my acknowledgements as those who have prayed, critiqued, encouraged and walked with me in this caregiving journey.

My son, Caleb – for his support and encouragement. He mows the lawn so I have time to write. He prays for me and never criticizes my calling to write – even if it interrupts his own schedule.

My sister, Kris Ediger and my brother, Phil Ediger – who have shouldered the primary role of caregivers for Mom.

The Saturday Sisters – a lifetime prayer group in Lawrence, Kansas. These sisters – Janet, Sharon, Ginger, Susan and Deb – lift me up, allow me to be real and provide chocolate when necessary.

My monthly critique group – wordsmiths who help me polish essays so the focus rings true and the nuggets of hope find a home. Thanks to Sally, Karen, Sara, Jane and SuZan.

Sally Jadlow – writer, chaplain and friend, who first told me about Create Space.

The followers of my blog – who encourage me with comments and help spawn new blog posts.

Nina Amir – author of "How to Blog a Book," which provided the impetus for this idea.

CrossRiver Media and Tamara Clymer – the publisher who saw

the value in a trilogy about Reverend G, novels where a woman minister, diagnosed with Alzheimer's, conquers her fear of forgetting God.

To the medical professionals who constantly research to find a cure for Alzheimer's Disease. May God grant them the wisdom to find it soon.

INTRODUCTION

The thief first appears as a slight blip on the memory screen – a word forgotten, a key chain misplaced and we laugh – at first.

Then more and more items are misplaced, numerous words forgotten until finally the very identity disappears. We no longer laugh because now we must seek out doctors who will tell us why Mother acts so strangely, why Father must no longer drive.

And then the dreaded diagnosis – dementia, Alzheimer's, the Long Goodbye.

The memory thief smirks. He has completed his work and left us bereft.

Sometimes they forget. And eventually, they no longer remember even those they birthed and raised.

How can we deal with these horrible changes in the dynamics of our families? How can we help our loved ones who sometimes forget?

And how can we take care of ourselves during the Long Goodbye?

This book is a collection of essays and meditations, to help the caregivers of loved ones who live out their final years, assaulted by the memory thief.

My hope is that this book will encourage you and help you realize you are not alone. May you find sustenance for your soul throughout its pages. May you know with a certainty that even if your mom or your dad, your sister or your brother no longer communicates with you – somewhere deep inside – their love for you remains.

May you find the grace to survive one more long and sad day.

But first … a bit of my family's history ….

He was a gentle man, this Mennonite farmer who lifted hay bales all day and threw them into a truck, then spent the evening softly strumming his guitar.

Henry, sometimes called Hank, was soft-spoken and so introverted that when he prayed or gave advice – everyone intently listened.

How I wish someone would have written down his wisdom, before he became forever silent.

I do own his Bible and sometimes – when I miss his quiet presence – I read through the verses he underlined:

"I create new heavens and a new earth; and the former shall not be remembered, nor come into mind" (Isaiah 65:17).

"The fear of the Lord is the beginning of knowledge; but fools despise wisdom and instruction" (Proverbs 1:7).

"But seek ye first the kingdom of God, and his righteousness; and all these things shall be added unto you" (Matthew 6:33).

He *did* seek the kingdom of God. Every morning, he read from his Bible and prayed for all of us. Every Sunday, he taught a class at church and made sure his family entered the doors in plenty of time to greet any visitors. He invited traveling missionaries home for a meal and asked them to tell their stories of lands across the sea.

And yet – not even his faith could save him from the memory thief.

Like a good farmer, he took care of the land and his home. On one cold November day, he lit a fire, but it didn't draw well. Having no heat in the house would be a problem. So he added fuel – a bit of kerosene to get it going. The fire leapt back on him, scorched the carpet in the living room, sparking flames on his wife's favorite chair.

He beat out the flames until he was sure everything was safe, then stumbled outside to gulp fresh air. That's where Mom found him, with his shirt hanging off his chest, deadly burns all over his body.

After four months in the hospital, several surgeries, daily debreeding sessions, graftings, sleepless nights, scars that roiled our stomachs, the acrid stench of putrified flesh – Dad was finally released. He returned home, unable to remember how the tractor made ruts in the plowed field or how to create chords on his guitar, why the cows didn't naturally come home without the gentle farmer gathering them in.

"Trauma-induced dementia," the doctors said. "Keep him at home as long as you can, but be prepared for a difficult journey."

My mother, the nurse, retired from her job. They moved from the farm to town, into a house that could accommodate a wheelchair if needed.

"I'll never put him in a nursing home," Mom said. She became his caregiver, daily, monthly, for ten long years.

My sister moved home to help. Together they fed him, bathed him, rolled him over when he graduated to the hospital bed. The silencing of his wise advice cut deeply into our lives, and my heart ached when I visited him.

We connected through music, so I sang to him. A spark would kindle in his eyes, especially for his favorite hymn, "Blessed Assurance."

Then one April, when the spring tulips erupted into bright yellow and purple blooms, when the promise of life budded everywhere – the spark disappeared. I knew it would not be long.

In May, he graduated to heaven. A release for all of us, especially for Dad. Sometimes death is a relief.

With her mate of 54 years buried, Mom devoted herself to volunteer work. She loved the grandchildren and followed their progress in school. She served meals to the hungry and counted Bingo cards at the nursing home.

One Thanksgiving, we each shared what we were thankful for. Mom's response, "I'm so glad I'm not in a nursing home – yet."

I wondered later if she had a premonition.

She began to misplace the pots and pans. She safety-pinned her house keys to the waistband of her pants, just in case she forgot how to get back into the house. She parked her car in the same spot at the grocery store so she could find it when she came out. She coped so well, it took us a while to figure out something was drastically wrong.

Then the questions began, "What day is it? What year is Caleb in school? Did we already have Christmas?"

My sister watched her, helped her, lived with her when she could have found her own apartment. I lived five hours away and noticed the changes even more readily than my siblings who saw her every day.

Then fainting spells, hard falls, congestive heart failure and a pacemaker. The doctor said, "She can't live independently anymore. Alzheimer's and an inoperable benign brain tumor."

We had already signed her up for a beautiful assisted living facility. But she fought us. "Why are you putting me here? There's nothing wrong with me."

We lied and hated ourselves. "It's only for a little while, Mom. Rehab after your pacemaker surgery. The doctor ordered it."

A partial truth is still a lie.

She's lived in assisted living for three years now. Confusion deepens. Her last living friends now reside in the memory care unit. No more trips to the mall to walk past stores and make fun of the clothes. No more biscuits and gravy at Braum's. No more crocheted projects. She sits quietly in her chair, sometimes in the dark, pretending to read – wishing she could comprehend the words.

Sometimes they forget and sometimes life forces them to forget. No matter what the situation or the health issue, caregivers are left to figure out a new normal – to somehow find hope and continue to love and live their own passions while dealing with this brutal disease.

We *can* find purpose in the Long Goodbye. We learn patience and strive for joy. We search for hope and treasure each moment we can still hold a hand, sing a hymn or stroke a forehead.

Sometimes they forget, but as long as *we* remember – their legacy continues.

May each of you, the caregivers, find some nugget to hang on to within these pages.

WHEN LIFE UNRAVELS

Sometimes writers struggle to find the right titles for their books. They highlight important words, search through a dictionary or wait until inspiration knocks at the door of their creative souls. Finally, amidst weeping and gnashing of teeth – they settle on a group of words that seems to tell their story yet also invites intrigue.

For my novel, "The Unraveling of Reverend G," the title floated through my brain just as easily as the first 20,000 words. I was so pleased my publisher, Cross River Media, decided to keep the title, because it seemed to state exactly what happens when Alzheimer's sets up its brutal residence in the brain. As the second and third books evolved, their titles also easily emerged. Thus, "Intermission for Reverend G" and "Final Grace for Reverend G" soon joined "The Unraveling of Reverend G" as a complete trilogy.

Someone recently asked me, "Why write about Alzheimer's? What caused you to choose that kind of story?"

It's a fair question. Over five million Americans struggle with the symptoms of dementia and/or Alzheimer's Disease. And with the progressive live-longer-and-fight-stronger attitude of the Baby Boomers, it is likely many of us will join that statistic. The numbers also indicate a whopping 30 million people are caregivers. Those stats make the topic both challenging and relevant.

The dictionary explains "unravel" as "to disengage or separate the threads of, to cause to come apart."

What a perfect visual of what happens to Alzheimer's patients! They gradually begin to disengage – from their passions, their routines and their families. As they lose the ability to remember faces or traditions, they shrink away from reality. They become separate from themselves, from the people they once were and the productivity they once enjoyed. They come apart. They unravel.

I saw this unraveling happen to my father and my mother. With Dad, speech unraveled until he spoke only the most basic of grunts. Then finally, even grunting disappeared as he forgot how to make sounds. With Mom, speech patterns remained lucid and clear, but her eyes held fear and her routines hid like shadows of the past.

In the Reverend G trilogy, the main character begins to unravel as the most commonplace joys change. She forgets a key word in the Lord's Prayer, and she begins to wonder when she will lose the names and faces of those she loves. Somehow, Reverend G finds joy in the everydayness of life although she secretly fears she may forget the Lord she serves. She unravels, yet all around her, people find encouragement through her bold desire to keep on trying.

Another definition of "unravel" gives me hope. This definition moves scientists forward "to resolve the intricacy, complexity or obscurity" of a subject, "to clear up or unravel a mystery."

That is my hope and the desire for every caregiver who puts in a 36-hour day. We long for someone, somewhere to unravel the mystery of Alzheimer's and make it go away.

The Alzheimer's journey reminds us that inside each person who sometimes forgets, resides a soul and some type of thought process. Connections may be flawed, but communication is still possible on some level – until the very end.

The Reverend G books and this current book needed to be written to remind caregivers to search for hope and to believe their incredibly difficult work has eternal significance.

As the author, Reverend G asked me to share her voice so readers could look differently at Alzheimer's victims and appreciate the people they once were – the souls they still are.

"Sometimes They Forget" is also a legacy to those people who so patiently care for those who forget. It is a mirror that reflects my own family – my dad who died within the shadows of dementia, my mother who fades away daily in the unraveling of Alzheimer's Disease.

But ultimately, I wrote this book because one day I woke up with a story in my head and characters who begged to escape.

And I wrote this book for you – to find encouragement, to learn from and to pass on so the next generation never forgets.

ASKING THE WHY QUESTION

Ever since the patriarch Job lived his troubled life, we have been asking "Why?"

Actually, the question "Why?" was probably asked since the beginning of time. Perhaps Adam halted in his naming of the animals to ask, "Why, God? Why did you spend so much time on the colorful details of the bluejay, then throw together this ridiculous version of the dodo bird? Was this your idea of a joke, some cosmic type of humor only you and the heavenly angels understand?"

The first mother, Eve, no doubt asked "Why?" as well. "Why, God? Why couldn't my sons find a peaceful way to work out their problems? Why did Cain have to take Abel's life? Why even allow me to birth these boys if you're just going to take one of them away, then condemn the other one to a life of exile? Why, God? Why?"

Every infertile woman, every family standing beside a coffin, every couple whose marriage ends in divorce at sometime in the process will ask, "Why?"

Those of us who watch the shadows of Alzheimer's dissipate the strength and fervor of a parent or a sibling or a beloved grandparent ask "Why? Why did this horrible disease choose our family? Why, God, have you allowed this to happen to us?"

We seek answers because we strive to make sense of this horrible thing that has happened. If we can somehow underscore the event with a logical answer, we can put together a plan for dealing with it.

But life doesn't work that way.

We cannot control the surprise ending of a vibrant life nor can we surround Alzheimer's with some sort of reasoning. Scientific researchers continue to search for its origins, but why it chooses one family over another, one sibling over the others – no one completely understands.

No earthly logic can explain why my mother lives within the shadows of the Long Goodbye. She has always been an active woman, working throughout the years as a registered nurse, caring for others. Involved in her church, she was strong in her faith. She exercised every day, walked the hallways briskly at her job and within the fences of our Oklahoma farmstead. She cooked nutritious meals and when research exploded about the danger of too many carbohydrates, she cut back on the pies, cakes and cookies. Her physical body at the age of 88 remains fairly healthy. It is only her brain that atrophies and betrays her.

Why? What is the key to this disease and how can we as a family somehow deal with it from the viewpoint of a logical answer?

We can't.

Like faith, we have to accept it as it is and believe a higher power will absorb the shock and give us the grace we need to care for Mom, even when we don't understand – *especially* when we don't understand.

But good old Job provides a possible solution to the dilemma, something I can hang on to when my fists are clenched in angry denial. The answer hides within a verse I discovered years ago when I asked God why my baby had to leave my womb at 12 weeks. This verse helps me confront the "Why" that whispers every time I visit Mom in the facility and miss the woman she used to be.

This verse is relevant only in the New American Standard version. Other versions don't even come close to answering Why. But here, in this one passage, lives three possible scenarios.

"Whether for correction, or for His world, or for lovingkindness – He causes it to happen" (Job 37:13 NASB).

For correction: Sometimes God allows terrible things to happen because we need to be shocked into reality and reminded he is sovereign. Perhaps in those moments of horrific happenings, we will reset our course and start over.

Did Adam and Eve raise Seth differently because of what they learned through their parenting of Cain and Abel? Didn't God remind the Israelites to stay away from foreign altars by allowing snake bites to kill and maim? Hasn't history taught us to be careful of the Hitlers of this world because of the Holocaust?

When terrible things happen to us, one response might be "What can I learn from this situation?" Rather than the "Why" question, rephrase it with "What?"

As gracious and loving as God is, he sometimes allows terrible things to happen. Why? So we can learn from our experiences and grow up.

For His world: We live in a fallen and depraved world. We are deceived into thinking we can fill their minds with pornography and not face any consequences. We believe we can speed and drive drunk and nothing will happen because we are somehow immortal. We eat what is not good for us, buy guns and forget to hide the bullets from children, look at someone's skin color and judge him.

Our world is not a safe place to live, so obviously – bad things are going to happen. Tornadoes, floods, earthquakes – all factor into the orb we inhabit. None of us avoids all tragedy during our lifetimes. It is part of the definition of living.

Why does God allow the world to turn against us? To remind us we are human and a better place *does* exist. Tornadoes will not touch heaven, nor will the sin of someone else force thorny consequences on families. Heaven and an eternal existence with God is something we long for, live for and hope for. This world will someday disappear. God wants to remind us he has planned for something better.

For lovingkindness: This seems to be the most difficult of the Job verse answers. Sometimes God allows certain tragedies to happen because he is a loving God. Is that backward, an opposite world sort of treatise? I do not believe we can ever second guess Almighty God.

But I do wonder… did God allow the groom to be killed the night before his wedding because he would someday betray his bride and destroy his family?

Does God invite little children into his heavenly arms instead of allowing them to live full lives because he knows their homes and their families will be bombed into oblivion and it is kinder to take them out of the horror?

Will God prevent one of his daughters from finishing a degree because he knows that pathway is the wrong direction for her?

I do not pretend to know what God determines about anyone else's life, but I do know he has sometimes worked his backward lovingkindness in my life. Hindsight is always wiser than the present experience.

God allowed me to be downsized out of a good job to force me to rest. Then he pointed me toward something better. Unemployment was hard, but the next job was so much better for me and fit my giftings. My "Why?" question became God's answer, "Just wait and see what I have for you."

How does Job 37:13 fit in with the journey of Alzheimer's?

Part of the answer has to include the world we live in. The stresses, the electromagnetic fields around us that affect our brains, the ways we have destroyed our food chains and polluted our water source, the chemicals we pour into our bodies that taste good but end up affecting the brain. All these worldly systems we have invented may contain a clue.

I hope God isn't correcting me or any of my family members by allowing us to watch Mom suffer. But I am willing to ask God to teach me through the process, to grow patience in me and hopefully – by sharing these words with you – to transfer hope within these pages.

I can't imagine how God would be showing his lovingkindness through this disease, unless he somehow wants to protect Mom from a future tragedy. She has no cognitive formulation of the world around her. She does not care who will become president in the next election. She is unaware of racial tensions, ISIS terrorists and a failing economy. She just wakes up every morning and shuffles to breakfast in the dining hall, then back to her room to turn up the television and wait for lunch.

Mom was a worrier throughout her life. Fear lived as a constant companion. But in her silent world of Alzheimer's, she has no cares, no worries. She lives in a protective globe and waits to be released to heaven when her timeline scrolls to the end. Perhaps God, in his lovingkindness, has gifted her with Alzheimer's so fear will no longer visit. He is protecting her from despair.

The question is "Why?" but the answer is "Who." God is in control of everything, and when we cannot understand – the best thing we can do – is run into his loving arms.

AN ETHICAL DILEMMA

The dilemma arises when a caregiver faces the ultimate decision. "Should we put our mother through a surgery, knowing it may save her life, but at the age of 88, it will only prolong her journey into Alzheimer's? What should we do?"

The decision, of course, ultimately rests with that family and the medical professionals, but it is a quandary many of us face as our parents age without the ability to express what they want for their own bodies.

This is one reason why families should have discussions about final wishes. Show your children where you keep the will and the life insurance papers. Finish paying for the memorial service and the preparation of the body so your children don't have to mess with difficult decisions while grief is fresh.

Medical professionals are trained to preserve life, to "do no harm." They are skilled in the various ways to test for disease, treat symptoms and perform surgeries that prolong life. Their protocol demands they do everything possible to save a life.

But at some point, don't we have to ask the hard questions? Is Alzheimer's any type of quality life? Would our loved ones want to go through the pain of surgery, the rehab after surgery and still face an even longer period of time living within the shadows of Alzheimer's?

My family faced this decision with Mom's pacemaker surgery. Her heart needed the extra stimulation because she was passing out, bumping her head and struggling with all sorts of physical problems. Doctors determined she needed a pacemaker, and the decision was made quickly by those who care daily for Mom.

No one thought to ask her, because she was in the Alzheimer's stage where decisions seem insurmountable. She couldn't decide to eat lasagna at the Olive Garden or a hamburger at McDonald's. Making a life-altering decision about a pacemaker fell completely out of her realm of possibilities.

So the family opted for extending her life and helping her breathe easier with a pacemaker. It was supposed to be an easy surgery, in and out in a couple of days.

But complications set in, and Mom's mental status quickly deteriorated from confusion to dementia. The end result was four days in the hospital with a transfer to nursing home care for rehabilitation.

During her stay in the hospital, the doctor observed her increased confusion and decided she could no longer live independently. After rehab, she would move to assisted living.

Fortunately, my siblings and I had seen the possibility of her final prognosis. We had already visited several facilities and found the one we felt Mom would like best. We were already on the list and able to seamlessly offer extended long-term care for our mother in a beautiful facility with caring professionals to help her.

But I wondered if we had made the best decision. Would it not have caused less harm to let Mom's brave heart just wear itself out and wing her to eternity where there is no pain, no surgeries and no Alzheimer's – forever and ever?

As I stayed night with Mom in the hospital, she experienced a rare moment of lucid thought and communication. She asked, "What did they do to me?"

I explained about the pacemaker and the complications of a collapsed lung, the possibility of pneumonia. "Your heart needed to be fixed, Mom," I said, glad for this moment between us but wishing we could be talking about something besides her difficult prognosis.

She raised up in bed, setting off monitors that blinked and brought nurses running. "If they would have asked me," Mom declared, "I would have said 'No.'"

A thousand shards of guilt pierced my soul. If we would have asked you.

But at that moment of decision, you weren't lucid. You weren't clear about what you wanted, what your desires for your own health involved. We let the medical professionals do their work, because we didn't know how else to keep you with us a few more months, a few more precious moments. We were afraid to let you go.

Ultimately, our decision to allow Mom's pacemaker surgery and the resulting complications condemned her to a longer lifetime of Alzheimer's. Even more months and as it turned out – more years – living in the shadows of cognitive decline and plaque-infested grief.

She would live in a beautiful facility, but the quality of her life would not continue. Giving up her independence weakened her spirit. She was angry, and rightly so. By saving her life, we had taken her soul-living away. We had denied her the freedom to live the rest of her days in her home, feeding the birds, walking around the yard and reading the paper at the antique kitchen table she restored.

When I arrived back in Kansas, the first thing I did was to instruct my son that absolutely no life-saving measures should be performed on me. "If I get Alzheimer's like Grandma, and if I'm not able to take care of myself, the best way you can love me is to let me go. Let me die. Please."

Then I wrote down my last wishes' papers and finalized everything in my will. Do no harm. Let me go.

In the third book of the Life at Cove Creek Series, "Final Grace for Reverend G," Jacob and Chris also faced this decision. Writing about this serious topic in a fictional story was easier than living through it with my mother. I knew what Reverend G would choose because I knew my own choice and what I felt was the sanest and kindest way to go.

As an author, I could manipulate my characters, use my research to anticipate decisions and foreshadow with a certainty that the story would support the plot. But real life is not a novel. Real life requires that we look at the lifetimes of our loved ones and determine what is best for them. If they have not given us clues or written down their wishes, then we have to listen to the professionals and choose wisely.

Sometimes we make the wrong choice.

My mother's heart continues to beat strong and pump the blood her system needs to support life. But her brain no longer responds to questions or conversation. Her body lives on, but her soul has shut down. Her personality has changed in the months since her surgery, and I wonder how much of that change is our fault.

When it comes to ethical dilemmas, I believe we must consider the overall character of our loved ones – what they have shared with us and what they have recorded in their last wishes.

For me, there is no debate. Choosing between a life of

Alzheimer's versus stepping into eternity is easy. I prefer heaven.

But each family has to make that choice for their loved one, and the journey of Alzheimer's demands we be prepared for such a question.

Now I pray that God will rescue Mom from this horrid disease before she becomes completely bedridden, medicated out of her mind and screaming with nightmarish fear. Ultimately, I also hope Mom will forgive us for agreeing with the doctor and prolonging her existence.

My encouragement to you is to talk with your loved ones while you can. Make certain you know their wishes for end of life decisions. And if possible – be strong enough to let them go.

ACTION POINTS AS LIFE UNRAVELS

Since life is so unpredictable, it often unravels. All our carefully constructed plans can fall apart within minutes. The doctor presents a frightening diagnosis. We open an email intended for someone else. The consultant decides our jobs are expendable – and so are we.

What do we do when life unravels? How do we react so that the very essence of our being fails to rupture?

Psalm 43 contains practical action points to help us when life unravels.

Action Point 1: Focus on God instead of the problem.

Psalm 43:1-2, "Vindicate me, O God, and plead my case against an ungodly nation; O deliver me from the deceitful and unjust man! For you are the God of my strength; why have you rejected me? Why do I go mourning because of the oppression of the enemy?"

God delivers us from oppression and pleads our case. As Mom's memories of me fade, I face a new and blatant form of oppression. How can a woman forget the child she birthed and raised?

Alzheimer's interferes with the circuits of memory. When I visit Mom and she looks at me as if she knows she should remember something, fails to place me in her mental archives, I feel that knee-jerk pain of rejection. When I mention Caleb, her grandson, she begins to fit the pieces together.

Oh, yes – you're Caleb's mother; therefore, you must be my daughter. I can't remember your name, but somehow I know you.

This is when I need God – someone stronger than I to plead my case and vindicate me.

When Mom asks me the same question over and over, I need God's patience to help me sit beside her and gently speak the same words. "It's Tuesday, Mom. February, 2016."

When we eat together in the dining room, and Mom cannot introduce me to the chef because she can't remember my name. When we stroll around the pond and Mom suddenly reverts to the angry statement, "You kids shouldn't have put me here." When we sit quietly in her room, reading books, and I know she isn't comprehending any of the words – these are the moments when I need God to be my support.

As I focus on God and his strength, I begin to think more positive thoughts and inch forward in baby steps toward accepting the next phase of Mom's illness.

Action Point 2: Focus on the lesson instead of the pain.

Psalm 43:3, "O send out your light and your truth, let them lead me; let them bring me to your holy hill and to your dwelling place."

God's light and truth lead me through the unraveling yarns of Mom's health issues. Even within the struggle of long-distance caregiving, he brings me to that place of utter peace, that inner holy of holies where I rest in his strength.

As I stay alert for his light and truth, he whispers the phrase of a song or directs me to a passage of scripture. When I focus on the lesson rather than the pain, God teaches me more of what I need to know in my faith journey. His beacon of truth points me to some of the richer treasures of faith and trust.

He reminds me that he has a greater purpose for my life and also for my mother's life. For some reason, she has been chosen to live through this Alzheimer's journey. And we – her children have also been chosen to show the world how it can be done.

We CAN focus on the lesson rather than the pain. We CAN encourage other residents and family members and help them know what to expect. We CAN be an encouragement to the health care providers who so patiently assist our mother each day.

As we focus on the lessons God wants to teach us, the pain of this journey becomes the secondary focus and a bit easier to bear.

Action Point 3: Focus on the future instead of the present.

Psalm 43:5, "Why are you in despair, O my soul? And why are you disturbed within me? Hope in God, for I shall yet praise him, the help of my countenance, and my God."

King David reminds us to stay in hope. I think of this important principle as, "Living in the Yet."

To live in the yet, I focus on the future – when this present circumstance wears down, when I work through the grief, when I learn the important lessons God wants to teach me.

Focus on the "yet" while I wonder how much longer this Alzheimer's will last. Focus on the place where Mom will be someday, happy in heaven, walking along with Dad and all her relatives and friends. So many of them already there and waiting for her to cross over.

Focus on the time when I will meet her there and she will know me without any prompting. She will remember her first-born and how she drove me to piano lessons, cheered for me at ballgames and worked hard to pay for my education.

All the unravelings of life, these temporary afflictions, eventually end. Some last longer than others and test our endurance. Some need extra amounts of God's power-filled grace. Some are blessedly brief. But all trials eventually end. All unraveling will come to the end of their source and lay in a heap on the ground or result in a beautiful project that glorifies the creator.

As we live in the yet, we learn to praise God that the end will indeed occur – in his timing. Then hopefully, our faith muscles will be stronger, our trust in him deeper.

No matter what unravels next, be grateful for Psalm 43 and determine to live in the yet.

THOUGHTS ABOUT PRAYER

Several readers of the Reverend G books have commented, "I really like how Reverend G prays. She just talks to God, like a regular conversation."

This comment encourages, but also saddens me. I think we've missed something.

Have we neglected to teach about conversational prayer in our churches? Do people not know prayer really is just talking and listening to God – having a conversation with the one who unconditionally loves us?

Have we presented God so fiercely as the High and Mighty One that we can't approach him on a personal basis – as if he is a judge who waits to zap us for wrong-doing and spawns fear in our souls?

Legalism paralyzes prayer.

God is indeed worthy of our respect and awe. He is the Alpha and the Omega, the Beginning and the End. He created each of us as a unique specimen of human DNA. He injected us with talents and gifts so each of his children could find a niche in life and glorify him.

He is the Creator who fashions a unique sunrise every morning and blankets the sky with orange and turquoise sunsets. He is the one who painted tiny white slivers on the tails of blue jays, then daubed great blobs of crimson on cardinals. He sees each of us swimming in our mothers' wombs, plans each day of our lives and decides which little girl will have curly hair and which tiny boy will sport dimples that wink when he smiles.

God is also Abba Father – Daddy God, the personal Divine who wants us to cling to him, climb up in his lap and love him back. He wants to hear our heart cries, even though he already knows them. Because when we cry out to him, it proves we need him and we believe he has enough strength to help us.

Prayer underscores our trust in God.

We can tell God exactly how we feel about life, because He knows our inmost emotions. He also knows our motives, so we can be honest and vulnerable enough to tell him when life sucks and we don't appreciate what we're going through and how we wonder why he doesn't do something about it.

And does God Almighty answer us? Of course he does. He is, after all, the Word – the one who communicates with his children on a personal level. But we have to learn how to listen to him, to find that still small voice inside our souls.

"In the beginning was the Word, and the Word was with God, and the Word was God" (John 1:1).

Words are the tools of communication. We can talk honestly to God and listen to him whenever and wherever we are, because he is always available, because he is the Word and therefore, he wants to communicate with us.

Reverend G has no special heart line to God. She's just like the rest of us, except she really is a fictional character. She teaches us that prayer is just a one-on-one heart connection between human beings and God, the one who created us and loves us completely and forever.

Like Reverend G, when life gets tough, we can genuinely state, "God, I can't stand it."

And he will understand, because sometimes Jesus couldn't stand it either. He rowed across the lake when too many people pummeled him with their needs. He decided to take a break. "God, I can't stand it."

Drops of blood leaked from his body before he marched to the cross. He was human and not exactly excited about the brutal execution he was about to endure. "God, I can't stand it."

The Spirit sits with us in Mom's room as she struggles to remember what day it is and how to tie her shoes – a task she patiently taught each of her three children. God watches and hears our cry, "God, we can't stand it."

Some prayers employ the beauty of the older English language, reminding us of ancient saints who read from the Psalter each day and used the oldest versions of the Holy Bible. Sweet words and ones we should revere.

But the greatest of prayers are those that strip us of any pretense and explode from the deepest places of need. When we can't even utter the words, "Dear God" or "Amen." Those prayers are the ones that simply hold out the need and trust God will listen and respond.

"We can't stand it, God. We need you."

THE POWER OF MUSIC

As the trauma-induced dementia stole my father away, one joy remained – the memories of music. Although he lost his ability to speak and to sing and he no longer strummed his old Gibson guitar or plunked chords on the piano, the memories of music remained.

I saw it in his eyes. Although Dad gradually lost the ability to respond by voice or even touch, the lyrics and the sounds of music cached in his shriveling brain. Eighth notes and rests, fermatas and repeat signs retained their sacred hold on Dad's soul. Although he loved many types of music - country western, classical and the harmonies of chorales – it was the hymns that evoked life to the very end.

Research has shown the prefrontal cortex and the cerebrum retain music even when other areas have begun to atrophy. The dimensions of music such as pitch, rhythm, timbre, melody and reverberation remain even as nouns , verbs and quality of speech disappears. These musical dimensions can remain as individual perceptions even if one or more of them begin to fade.

My dad was no longer able to physically exhibit rhythm yet melodies somehow remained intact. His favorite hymn became our way to connect, the one gem of communication that held our hearts together even as his dementia progressed.

Whenever I entered Dad's bedroom at the end of the hallway, I started singing this old hymn. Since the day he gave his heart to Jesus, during halftime of a college basketball game, the blessed assurance of his salvation wrapped his heart in security. Dad chose this hymn whenever given a chance during sing-alongs. He and I sang it together when we ministered on Sunday afternoons at the city mission. He carried that blessed assurance with him even during the tragic fire that started his long road toward dementia. Dad's soul wrapped itself around the meaning of those words and blessed him during the darkest times.

"Blessed assurance, Jesus is mine. Oh what a foretaste of glory divine.
Heir of salvation, purchase of God. Born of his spirit, washed in his blood.
This is my story, this is my song. Praising my Savior all the day long.
This is my story, this is my song. Praising my Savior all the day long."

As I sang through all three verses of his hymn, I stroked Dad's hair and patted his hand. A spark lit up his eyes. Somewhere inside that ravaged brain, the music stirred a memory. Although he could not verbally share it with me, his eyes spoke the truth. The blessed assurance of his eternal security in Christ still existed. His soul echoed the joy of an inward praise to his Savior.

During Easter weekend of 2004, I once again entered Dad's bedroom and sang his hymn. I patted his hand and looked into his eyes for that familiar spark of remembrance. But this time, it was gone. Only a blank stare greeted me. The dementia had finally stolen from him the last vestige of music. I knew Dad was on his way to heaven where songs would never end.

One month later, my sister called me and said. "Dad's finally Home. It's over."

At his funeral, we once again sang the words to "Blessed Assurance." The music reverberated throughout the sanctuary, surrounded his dear body lying in the coffin and echoed through the hallways of the church. As Dad's earthly story ended, that blessed assurance became his epilogue. His song carried him into the arms of Jesus and once again, I marveled at the power of the music.

As caregivers, we must discover those special songs that comfort our loved ones. As we sing the melodies or play an instrument at the bedside, we connect once again. And in that connection, we find joy even in the waning moments of life. The power of the music transcends our one-dimensional lives and transports us all to the spiritual haven we long for.

Even now, all three verses come easily to mind and whenever I sing them, I remember the gentle man who understood the power of music.

I love you, Dad, and I miss you. In your memory, I continue to sing your song.

SEVEN TIPS FOR CAREGIVERS

When life unravels into Alzheimer's and/or dementia, it is vitally important for caregivers to carry survival tools. When we implement these tools, it helps us survive the process of caregiving and encourages us to keep going for the long term. These seven tips can restore hope and sanity.

Tip # 1: Talk to Me

It is easier and sometimes more comfortable to talk around someone who has Alzheimer's rather than to try and engage them in conversation. Since they can't always respond, we sometimes forget they're even in the room. But on some level, they want to communicate with us and especially in the earlier stages of the disease – they will know when we are ignoring them. We need to look at our loved ones, smile and talk to them.

One lovely spring day, my sister and I drove Mom to the emergency clinic. She had a vicious cough, followed by a wheeze so we were worried about pneumonia or some other sort of lung problem. In the examination room, Mom sat on the sterile table while the doctor discussed her symptoms with my sister and me. Mom listened and acted alert, but we talked around her.

At that time, I was in the middle of editing my book, writing about Reverend G and how others ignored her because she struggled with aphasia and could no longer communicate. I suddenly realized what we were doing to our own mother. I stood up, looked directly at Mom and said, "The doctor is going to give you some medicine. It will help your cough. What do you think about that?"

In her typical take-charge fashion, she announced, "I'm fine. Just fine. Nothing wrong with me."

In spite of Mom's rebuttal, we drove to the pharmacy and bought the medicine. She swallowed it and within a few days, the wheezing had disappeared and she seemed to feel better. On my drive back to Kansas, I was relieved to have given her the opportunity to state her opinion. Hopefully within that moment, she felt as if we had not forgotten her.

The character of Reverend G would remind us, "Keep communicating with me, even if I can't answer. Look me in the eyes, touch me, show me you still care about the person hiding inside me. Remind me that I still matter. Talk to me."

Tip # 2: Don't Argue with Me

When memory loss or paranoia sets in, we may find ourselves marching into a debate. But arguing with an Alzheimer's victim is pointless. They always win.

Instead of arguing back and forth, ask pertinent questions. By forcing our loved ones to think about the questions, we may together figure out a solution.

With her paranoia, Mom often makes up the most elaborate stories. And if she dreams something, she believes it truly happened. "Someone came into my house and stole my checkbook. Then the robber took it to the bank, forged my signature and stole all my money."

This story was of course, ludicrous, but it did not help to say, "No, Mom. That didn't happen." She was convinced the story was real, so we argued back and forth about this phantom criminal,

"That didn't happen, Mom."

"Yes, it did."

"No, it didn't."

Instead of arguing, ask questions. "Now, Mom, how do you think this person broke into the house? No doorknobs have been broken. No windows are shattered. And how did this person forge your signature when he doesn't really know you and can't copy your style of writing?"

As I asked questions, Mom was forced to consider the answers rather than the arguments. Although she no longer had the ability to find reasoning in hypothetical situations, just the presence of a question caused her to pause and ended the debate. After considering a few questions, she forgot all about the story – until she brought it up again. Then we started all over with more questions.

Asking questions can also divert the conversation to another subject. For several months, Mom was concerned about someone stealing her clothes. None of us in the family wears the same size as Mom and none of her clothes fit the styles we wear, but she was convinced we were coming into her room at night and stealing some of her favorite clothes.

So when she told me, "I can't find that sweatshirt. Someone stole it," I diverted the conversation to something complete different by using a question.

"Do you like that plant in the window, Mom, or would you rather I move it over in the corner?"

She was forced to answer my question and for a while, she forgot all about the stolen clothes.

It takes a bit of practice and perseverance to ask questions instead of arguing. But arguments do nothing to solve the problem and only bring more frustration to both parties. Open-ended questions help everyone settle down so our visits are more productive and enjoyable.

Who of us wants to spend our precious time debating when we need to spend whatever remaining time we have just loving each other? It's a better use of time to acknowledge our loved ones have a legitimate concern, treat them with respect and ask a few questions.

The Golden Rule of Alzheimer's is: Treat your loved ones the way you want to be treated in fifty years.

Tip # 3: Keep Laughing

It is a well-documented fact that laughter helps us survive the struggles of life. Laughter releases healthy endorphins and gives us a sense of well-being. Throughout the 36-hour days of Alzheimers, laughter may be the only thing that helps us survive.

My mother, an avid reader, goes to library and Hospice book sales and buys stacks of books. Then she returns home and reads the same book several times. She has forgotten she read that particular book, so she turns the pages over and over, laughs at the same sections and solves "Who done it" mysteries. Then she returns her books for another stack and reads one of those over and over. Our family laughs about Mom's funny reading quirk.

As farmers, my family feeds and butchers a beef every year. Then we divide the meat so all of us have fresh beef for several months. One year, my mother called me and said, "Come get half my meat. I don't need all of this."

So I drove to Oklahoma, loaded up my cooler with fresh beef and covered it with ice. I stocked my freezer, made wonderful hamburgers for my son and thanked God for the provision.

About a month later, my mother called. "I'm going to put a lock on my freezer. Someone has stolen half my meat."

"Mom, you gave me half your meat."

"I know that, but someone has stolen half of it." My son and I laughed about that incident for months.

Although much of Alzheimers and dementia causes brutal sadness, some incidents can be funny. But we may have to search for the humor. For example, parents who can't hear yet refuse to wear hearing aids. In the middle of a restaurant, Mom shouted her order. Since she couldn't hear herself well, I guess she thought speaking louder would help.

My teenaged son laughed when Grandpa started cursing. Words he had never uttered before suddenly slipped out of his mouth. The same words I would not allow my son to say were now acceptable from Grandpa's dementia-clouded voice.

When women in their eighties suddenly enjoy sleeping with stuffed animals, it's kind of funny. When Mom puts her pants on backwards or leaves curlers in her hair for church – we have to laugh.

Remember and treasure the funny things your loved ones say or do. Journal about them or share them with support groups. Laughter will help you endure another 36-hour day. Find the humor in the situation and keep laughing.

Tip # 4: Remember the Life Story

Each of us has a life story and while we're living it, we often don't realize how important it is. The life story defines us, leaves a legacy and tells our loved ones who we were and how we dealt with each day and each situation.

For the caregiver, the life story becomes vital. As we remember the life story, we find clues for how to deal with our loved ones and ease their anxiety.

During her life, did she like animals? Then we need pet therapy. Find a dog or cat she can pet and cuddle and a facility that welcomes pets. Or find pictures of pets and hang them around the room. Make her environment more comfortable by including the animals she once loved.

Did he enjoy watching the sunset? Then watch it together every night, and especially – when he seems agitated. Develop a routine around sunsets and find pictures you can share with him on nights when the clouds obscure God's colorful panorama.

Was she in the military? Maybe she would enjoy hearing military songs such as "Anchors Away" or "From the Halls of Montezuma." Record them and play them when you visit.

My mother was a nurse, so when she's anxious—we use medical jargon. "Remember, Mom, when you were a nurse and you wanted your patients to take their medicine? Well, you need to do that now. Swallow your meds."

When Mom doesn't want to do something, we ask the doctor to write a prescription. She's accustomed to obeying doctors' orders. The doctor wrote a script that stated, "Arlene is no longer able to drive a car." Mom didn't like it, but she obeyed because the authority of doctors was an imperative part of her medical training.

Dad loved sports, so even when he couldn't comprehend which

team was playing, we turned on the television and watched ballgames together.

Is your loved one a Bible lover? Read scripture when you visit or buy an audio version of the Bible so she can listen to it when she feels alone.

Did she love professional manicures? Many assisted living facilities have a nail salon. Bless her by giving her this gift.

As we remember the life stories of our loved ones, we are also reminded to write our own memoirs. Start working on your life story and get it in print so your children will know how to communicate with you. Leave a legacy by supplying the clues that will help others know your life stories. It will be a lasting memorial and vital, if you become one of those who sometimes forgets.

Tip # 5: Take Care of Yourself

Healthcare professionals emphasize the importance of caregivers taking care of themselves. Up to 70% of caregivers experience the clinical symptoms of depression. In 20% of caregivers, their health deteriorates, they suffer with some type of chronic illness and sometimes they die before the Alzheimer's patient. The caregiver's immune system is impacted up to three years after their loved one dies.

One of my friends took care of her mother for a two-week vacation. Immediately after she waved goodbye at the airport, she broke out in shingles. The doctor told her the culprit was stress.

We can't sit beside the bed day after day without a respite. We'll go crazy. We need to take a break.

We can utilize the daycare centers for Alzheimer's patients and share our struggles within support groups. We may need to spend time with a therapist to deal with our own emotions and the various stages of grief. We need short vacations and long vacations, and we need to take them without packing a bunch of guilt.

Remember how our parents left us with babysitters so they could have a night out? The roles are now reversed, and we need to do the same. Take a break. Schedule a free night on your calendar.

Try some of these suggestions:

- Walk through a rose garden and thank God for all the varieties he created.
- Browse through a quaint little bookstore, pet the store cat and buy a book – then take the time to sit down and read it.
- Observe the Sabbath and share a meal with friends.
- Spend time alone and do nothing.
- Color or try a new art project.
- Go to a movie and munch on the popcorn that isn't good for us.
- Watch a funny video.
- Enjoy the sunset and thank God for his orange and turquoise sky.

If your loved one is in need of care that you can no longer supply, find the right facility and arrange for the best professional care. Again, don't pack any guilt.

One of my friends cared for her husband for 16 years. Finally, when she celebrated her 81st birthday, she told her children she could no longer take care of Dad. They understood and agreed. Then, with her witty sense of humor, she reminded her family, "I don't do windows or guilt."

None of us want our children to feel burdened or to grow sick because of the stress of care. So … take care of yourself.

Tip # 6: Forgive Me

None of our loved ones planned to develop dementia or Alzheimer's. If they could cognitively understand, they would hate what the disease has done to our family. They would want us to forgive them. If they could communicate, they might speak some of these phrases:

"When I can't remember your name, but somehow your face looks familiar, please – forgive me."

"When I'm screaming at the nurse because I'm afraid, please – forgive me."

"When I keep begging to go home and you won't let me because you know it isn't wise, please – forgive me."

"When I make up stories about you that I think are true, please – forgive me."

"When I'm cursing at you and you're surprised I even know those terrible words, please – forgive me."

"When I throw my food or act like a toddler, please – forgive me."

"When you have to change my diaper, please – forgive me."

"When I ask you to repeat something, be patient. Remember when I read the same story to you over and over and over? Do that for me now and please – forgive me."

"Remember inside the deepest part of my soul, where the sacred meets the human and becomes eternal – I am really the same, loving person. Please – forgive me."

"I really DO know who you are, but right now – there's a shadow between us and I can't find my way through it. Please – forgive me."

"I love you with every fiber of my being, but I can't say the words any more. Please – forgive me."

"I ask you to understand and once again, please – forgive me."

Tip # 7: Pray

When the 36-hour day blends into the next, pray. When you need extra patience, pray. When you can't bear watching the symptoms of this horrid disease, pray.

While Dad was in the hospital recuperating from his burns, I often read scripture to him and then we prayed together. Just being close and calling on God, helped him make it through the night and strengthened me as I struggled to watch his suffering.

The best times of prayer are when we simply talk to God – no special vocabulary, no legalistic rules or regulations of religion – just an honest speaking that comes from the core of our souls.

We can learn how to listen for God's response, because he is within us. Deep within our souls, this sacred presence resides and God whispers his truth, "I am with you. I love you. I will help you."

As a loving father, he enjoys hearing our prayers and wants to communicate with us. He operates as the great physician who understands how the physical body works. He sees the plaque-infested brains of our loved ones and how the systems have skewed. He knows exactly what we're dealing with as caregivers of these precious loved ones.

He wants us to share our deepest thoughts with him: *God, I hate this disease and what it has done to our family. I can't stand it, God, not another minute. Do something and hurry up!*

He understands our frustration, our sorrow, our pain and our confusion when this beloved family member no longer knows how to love us. He hears the heart cries of people who come to him in emergency rooms, in the intensive care units and in the quiet rooms of assisted living facilities. He is able to do more than we ask because he knows exactly what is needed.

So when you are beyond your human resources and when you are so tired, you can't remember your own name – pray. When the grief of losing the very essence of who your parent once was grips you with a physical pain – pray.

When you don't know how to take the next step for the best care of your loved one – pray. When you need relief and release – pray. When the facility calls and asks you to come find your mother because she has wandered away – pray.

And as you pray, know God hears you. He will send strength, encouragement and his presence to help you.

SPEAKING THROUGH THE TEARS

Every time I am invited for a speaking event, this happens. I have learned to take Kleenex with me.

Someone in the audience either reaches for a tissue or wipes their tears away. Sometimes, from the people in the front rows, I see tears puddle in their eyes.

Maybe tears gather because my topic is centered around my mother's Alzheimer's and my father's dementia.

Maybe the grief is fresh because I include poignant stories about life on the farm and the way our family dynamics changed as our parents aged.

Maybe the truth causes tears because so many of us have experienced a life that unraveled. We need hope, and sometimes that hope hides behind layers of grief. Once the tears wash away denial, hope settles in. Even Jesus cried, and he was a mighty strong man.

Someone once told me that when I speak, I touch hearts. Their hearts leak and the result is tears.

I want to share hope and encouragement with caregivers and their families. I want my audience to understand as difficult as Alzheimer's and dementia are, researchers are working on ways to detect it earlier and possibly ward off the long-term effects.

I want caregivers to understand the only way to cope with this horrid disease is to hang on so tightly to God not even plaque in the brain will dislodge his grace.

Perhaps the people in my audiences cry because they need a venue where they can grieve the unraveling of their lives. We stay so busy doing the urgent we sometimes forget how important it is to grieve our losses – whether those losses come from death, from the destruction of a formerly-active brain or from a devastating diagnosis.

So I encourage you to bring on the tears and let them flow. Be honest and vulnerable enough to grab a Kleenex and wipe those puddles from your eyes.

Once you let those blocks of grief into the fresh air, you will discover hope waiting for another day.

REMINDER TO GIVE

One Christmas, I drove to Oklahoma to visit my relatives and celebrate the holiday. At a rest stop, I filled up my mug with chai tea, then stretched my legs and browsed through the gift shop.

On a swivel display, several colorful magnets stood out. One in particular, made me think of Mom. It was a pansy, the purple variety with a yellow center, the pansy Oklahoma grows in the early spring, a pansy like the ones in Mom's flower garden.

Pansies live through the blustery winters, then push their brave heads through frozen soil in mid-March. They remind us we can survive even the coldest of experiences and look forward to the warmth of a new season.

Mom, my sister and I have always planted and nurtured pansies and their cousins, the violas. They remind us to hang on to hope and now – during this season of Alzheimer's – pansies represent treasured memories of Mom's garden and her puttering around in the dirt.

I knew Mom would love this pansy magnet. I could imagine her placing it on her fridge next to the magnets that held pictures of the grandkids in their various growth stages.

But I hesitated. It was $2.50 for a tiny pansy magnet. Was it really worth that? No, probably not. Whoever created this "treasure" surely over-priced it. I could use that $2.50 for a nice protein bar that would help keep me alert and focused on the drive.

I decided to think about it. Maybe I would buy it on the return trip, then mail it to Mom or give it to her for Mother's Day.

But I should have listened to that inner nudge. I should have told myself, "To heck with your stupid budget and trying to live on pennies. Buy it now while you can."

But I didn't listen. I swished through the revolving door of the rest stop, drove on down the road, sipped my chai tea and forgot all about the magnet. Four months later when I drove to Oklahoma for the Easter break, I stopped at the same rest stop. I refilled my cup with iced tea, stretched my legs and browsed through the gift shop.

Suddenly I remembered the display of magnets, but they no longer decorated the shelves. No pansies, no flowers, no pretty magnets of any kind.

I still kick my inward self for not buying that magnet for Mom on that long ago trip. It was only $2.50, for pete's sake. Every time I drive to Oklahoma, I stop at the same rest stop and buy a cup of hot chai or refill my iced tea. I stretch my legs and browse through the gift shop, because that is what I do on my trips home. And every time, I remember what a small yet important gift that pansy magnet might have been to Mom.

For that season of time, perhaps she would have felt honored and loved. Maybe it would have given her a special something to focus on during the winters of forgetfulness when she knew something was wrong and she was afraid. Perhaps she would have touched it with longing and remembered the first-born daughter who lives so far away. Surely that kind of treasure is worth much more than $2.50.

Even if the gift shop begins to restock the pansy magnets, Mom no longer lives in her house. She has no refrigerator in her assisted living apartment. No place to put magnets that would give her a few moments of pleasure. She lives in a different season and probably has no recollection of the pansy plants she carefully placed in the ground and nurtured each year.

Gifts to others are never wasted. Life is short and it sometimes changes drastically from one day to the next. An email message that ends a job. A surprise diagnosis that triggers fear. Moving a loved one out of their home and into a facility.

Although it is important to stick to a budget and be frugal with our incomes, a giving heart is even more important – especially for those we love whose time on earth is limited.

So learn from my experience. Buy the stupid magnet or the plastic toy or a drink for a fellow traveler. Be a giver, because it's easier to spend a bit of money than to forgive yourself later.

CHOICES FOR ONE ROOM

"Your mother can no longer live independently," the doctor told us. He adjusted Mom's chart and fingered the stethoscope hanging around his neck. He seemed as nervous as the three of us, standing outside Mom's hospital room and trying to fathom this final prognosis. "It's time to consider some type of assisted living arrangement. I'll prescribe all her meds and the nurses in the facility will make sure your mother has everything she needs."

Assisted living is a nicer, somewhat softer tone for what Mom and her generation have considered the dreaded "nursing home." It's a final judgment on a life that no longer exists outside four walls, a stripping of freedoms and independence. No more driving to the grocery store to pick up whatever you need. No more puttering around the house or digging in the garden. Life is now devoted to one room or the sharing of space by residents locked within the same Alzheimer's shadows.

As we toured the various options, we discovered beautiful settings and professional staff who knew how to care for their residents and tried to meet emotional as well as physical needs. One place proudly sported a garden where Mom could have watched flowers poke their heads through early spring soil, but the room was so tiny and painted an ugly taupe. We knew she would hate it.

Another facility favored a homey atmosphere with a kitchen and dining hall in the middle and all the rooms attached like cubicles connected to an umbilical cord. Professionally decorated and only a few blocks from Mom's home, it seemed a good option until the director told us the price – well above our limit.

Finally, we toured the place where Mom once served as a volunteer with an almost prophetic aura of who Mom used to be. The rooms were spacious and the hallways wider than most facilities. Several choices for dining and living areas as well as a pond to walk around with ducks swimming serenely from shore to shore. The big advantage for this facility was that when the time came, Mom could easily be transferred to the Memory Care unit and we wouldn't have to find another place to completely uproot her.

So my sister and brother – who have power of attorney – signed the papers and we moved forward. Mom needed a couple of weeks in nursing home rehab, so that made it easy to tell her, "The doctor says you have to be here a couple of weeks." When those weeks ended, we told her again, "The doctor says you have to be here a couple of weeks." We repeated that same phrase for several months. At that point, Mom had no conscious awareness of time and although it seemed as if we were lying, it was the only way to help her embrace contentment until her room in the assisted living wing was ready.

What do you choose when your entire life and all your possessions are downsized to one room? We had to consider the various pieces of furniture that best fit the space and accessories to help Mom feel most comfortable in her new surroundings.

Family pictures of course, artfully displayed on the corner cabinet that belonged to her aunt. A small dresser, big enough to store her clothes yet serve as a TV stand. The daybed from Mom's guest room with her favorite quilt to keep her warm and provide extra color. An antique lamp I gave her with a crystal shade that reflected prisms of light. Her recliner. Some plants my sister repotted. Although Mom's room included a small kitchenette, we wanted her to eat the nutritious food in the dining room. So her dishes remained in the kitchen cabinets at her house. Later – we hoped much later – we would decide what to do with them.

Her walk-in closet and combination bathroom were bigger than any closets in my house, so it felt good to arrange Mom's clothes and hang them with the one-fourth inch separation of hangers she liked. Even in assisted living, it's important to consider the routines and habits of a lifetime. Try to make it seem like home, even though a part of you wants to scream about the injustice.

One day as I poured out my heart to God about Mom's situation, I looked around my own house. What would I choose to live with if I had only one room? Besides the basics of a bed and a dresser, what would give me the most joy? Pictures of my son, of course, but which of the many albums would I choose? The ones that remind me of the sweet baby I held or the albums memorializing his school years, the funky cowlick in his hair and the missing front teeth, the adolescent growth that foreshadowed the man he would become? What about his graduation pictures? Could I somehow condense my son's entire life into one album?

Which of my clothes would I choose? Certainly, I could not keep all my colorful scarves and jewelry, and I would miss those accessories. I love my kitchen dishes and how they coordinate in deep maroons, yellows and sage greens. But like Mom, I probably wouldn't need them.

And which of the shoes would I take? My boots are as much a part of the winter season as the snowflakes that float from the Kansas sky. Which of my colorful sandals that show off carefully pedicured toes? Which Bible of the many translations standing in regal importance on my shelves? How would I continue to write without all my files, my special desk and the pictures of Santa Fe that surround my office? And if I cannot write, how will my soul live?

I would want my pottery to remind me of the Southwest, those special pieces I found in unique stores in Taos and even in the Goodwill in Olathe, Kansas. Where would I store those terracotta pots and the vines that draped from their mouths? If I had no room for shelving, how could I enjoy the colors and textures I loved so much?

What of the many books that lined my office, lay in crooked stacks in my bedroom and piles on the kitchen table? These books waited for me to read their words, to marvel in the phrases and sentences of whoever claimed their authorship. I love books, the texture of their covers and the intense pleasure of turning another page. How could I possibly live without them?

I suppose within the shadows of dementia and Alzheimer's none of these items matter anymore. But every time I play my piano, open a book or wash a dish—I am grateful for how I still enjoy my things – my particular stuff. Who knows how long those treasures will last.

Mom was never a woman of material things. Her only collectibles were an armoire filled with Fostoria dishes and cups. When Dad entered the world of dementia, Mom sold her entire collection and the armoire then deposited the money in savings to help for Dad's future care. Not one dish is left, and somehow – even though her style is not mine – the loss sears me with a hidden grief.

As we settled Mom in her room, she seemed unaware of the new space, uncaring that her car was gone, her dishes absent and the cat who settled on her lap no longer a comforting warmth. Somehow, our grief at this stage in her journey seemed slightly assuaged by the attempts we made to keep her comfortable – to surround her with a semblance of past joy.

Months later, Mom asked, "Why am I in the nursing home? Why

did you kids do this to me?"

The stab of condemning guilt nearly knocked me over, and I blinked back tears. "The doctor said you could no longer live alone, Mom, and all of us have to work. We can't take care of you all day every day, so this is the best option. This is just a season of your life."

She rocked for a few minutes, then peered at me over her bifocals. "I don't like this season."

"Neither do I, Mom. Neither do I."

SEVEN HOLIDAY TIPS

How should we deal with our loved ones during the holidays? What are best practices to help those living with Alzheimer's enjoy these family reunions?

The calendar reminds us Thanksgiving is only a few weeks away and soon after comes Christmas. As much as we enjoy the family time, the abundance of good food and the reminders to be thankful – we also have to remember how stressful this time can be – especially for someone who suffers from Alzheimer's or dementia.

So here are seven tips to remember as you move into the holidays:

Don't expect your loved one to prepare any food.

One year, Mom tried to figure out a recipe to bring to our Thanksgiving meal. She wanted to feel as if she was still part of the festivities. "I'm not dead yet," she said, squaring her shoulders and marching into the kitchen. But she didn't realize what the process would involve. She worried about buying the groceries, had a difficult time making decisions about the size of the pan or the right ingredients and she kept losing the recipe.

We wanted her to feel connected to the process of cooking and bringing food to our celebrations, but it seemed too much of an effort. As we watched her struggle to find pots and pans, then wonder if she had made her salad – hundreds of times over – we realized it was time to stop expecting Mom to cook for the holidays. Even when she wanted to make something, we told her, "It's already taken care of, Mom. You don't have to worry."

At some point, participation becomes more of a struggle than a treasure.

If your loved one wants to shop for gifts, plan ahead.

Shopping, especially for the grandkids, is a pleasure few of us would deny our loved ones. But as dementia or Alzheimer's begin to manifest, even something as pleasurable as walking through the toy store can be a problem.

Be prepared with a shopping list and know the easiest way to enter and exit stores. Shop only in familiar places. New routines often bring discomfort. Forget about Black Friday shopping or the busyness of big box stores. Too many people jostling and too much noise may become a fearful experience.

Be patient, take plenty of time and be prepared to answer many questions. If possible, buy everything in one store.

At the checkout, carefully watch your loved one. Dealing with money may become a problem. Although Mom did well counting bills and coins, writing a check soon became a confusing activity. Be prepared for some battles regarding money issues. Especially in Mom's generation, saving money and choosing when to spend it became its own demographic.

If the money issue becomes too much of a battleground, leave the purchases and go home. Your loved one will soon forget about it. Better yet, shop online and have everything delivered.

During meals, include some of your loved ones' favorite foods.

My mom always wants pecan pie – for any holiday: Thanksgiving, Christmas and Easter. But none of the cooks in our family makes a decent pecan pie, although I've tried numerous times. So every year, my brother provides the Cool Whip and I buy a pecan pie. We cut the first piece for Mom. When it's time for her memorial service, we'll plan on the family meal including pecan pies.

Do an activity together, such as looking through Christmas cards.

Holding something concrete, feeling the texture and looking at the colorful pictures helps fill the time waiting for the ham to finish baking. Remind your loved one about the people in the pictures or tell a favorite story about the person who sent the card.

Be prepared to look at the cards several times during the holidays and repeat the same stories.

Encourage the grandchildren to make a special card for Grandma and tape it to her door or on one of the walls in her room. Every time you visit, talk about the card and remind her how much the grandchildren love her.

If you check your loved one out of assisted living for the day, be sure to check back in before dark.

As the sun sets, Alzheimer's patients often experience Sundowner's Syndrome. They may pace, say the same words over and over and exhibit anxiety. They feel safer in their rooms before dark, so make sure you time your meals and activities accordingly.

An Easter egg hunt or opening Christmas presents may become too long of an activity for Grandpa. Be alert for anxious or fearful symptoms and physical cues of distress.

The amount of time Grandpa can endure out of the facility gradually decreases. Begin to plan holiday activities at the facility. Most assisted living dining rooms will reserve a space for you and sometimes prepare the meals. Focus on whatever makes your loved one most comfortable. Spend an hour or so at the facility, then you can go back home and celebrate the rest of the day together.

If you travel for the holidays, it is not a good idea to include your loved one.

Traveling out of her comfort zone is difficult when Grandma struggles with dementia or Alzheimer's. Several hours cramped in a car or a plane, strangers everywhere, noise, unfamiliar surroundings, different types of foods and smells – all these issues can become a problem. Also consider the issues of health such as incontinence, medicines and special diets.

It makes more sense to hire a caregiver and let your loved one stay home or in the facility. When travel becomes an issue, determine that all holiday celebrations will be spent with Grandma, within her comfort zone. After she passes, you'll have more options.

What should you buy for the Alzheimer's patient?

Think about the regression your loved one is experiencing. At what age level is she now? Buy her a stuffed animal, a baby doll or a new pair of pajamas.

Put together an album of family members with childhood photos inserted next to their adult photos. This will help her recognize who they are now, because she remembers the children they once were.

Does she have a favorite piece of candy? Is she still able to enjoy eating at her favorite restaurant? Consider a gift card.

A comfortable sweater helps to keep her warm, but be prepared in case she loses it. Maybe she would like a new pillow or a colorful afghan to drape over her lap.

Be careful about the wrappings of presents. Figuring out how to break through Scotch tape may cause anxiety, and ribbons become a puzzle. A gift bag is easier. Help her fish through the tissue paper and find the gift.

One Christmas, I gave Mom a wooden cross, made in New Mexico and painted in her favorite colors. We hung it on her wall under the portrait of Jesus. For every holiday, I included a bag of her favorite Lifesaver mints which she hid in one of her drawers and always offered visitors.

Every year, I gave her a hug and a kiss, knowing the next Christmas might be completely different – another stage further into the shadow land of Alzheimer's.

For this current year, she still knows who I am, and I am grateful. Next year – maybe not.

SHADOWS OF ALZHEIMER'S

The shadows of autumn leaves dance across the Venetian blinds in my office. I enjoy this extraordinary moment of now.

With the changing of the season, I revel in the colors and textures – reds, oranges, golds – blended with the green leftovers of summer. The crunch of tiny acorns under my walking shoes, a pubescent pinecone that fell too early. Orange pumpkins reign over the steps next to my almost-withered summer annuals.

These are the sights and sounds of the autumnal season, often referred to as harvest season.

In the Reverend G books, the brave little minister wonders how to deal with her own shadows of Alzheimer's – the seasons that come and go, leaving her a bit more confused, a bit closer mentally to her younger self even as her physical body ages. She yearns to share her faith with the residents at Cove Creek yet she can't quite remember how to speak the Gospel.

In one of my favorite scenes in "Final Grace for Reverend G," she tries to preach a sermon and jumbles the story in an endearing yet tragic attempt to share her faith. What a character she is and how bravely she tries to deal with this disease that has stolen even the memory of ministry from her!

Surely the Lord God is with me and will not let his servant tremble with fear.

And yet I am somewhat fearful of what may lie ahead. Although I have faithfully served God within my congregation all these years...although I have spoken about faith often and forcefully from the pulpit, still – I am human and wonder what lies ahead.

God has not blessed me with the gift of prophecy but he is starting to warn me. Every morning when I open my Bible, I ask him, "Dear Father, what would you like me to read today? What will you teach me on this lovely morning?"

For the past four mornings, he has repeated the same instruction, "Isaiah 43:2-3."

"Really? Again? So here I am, reading the same passage and jotting down thoughts in my journal, asking you, sweet Holy Spirit, to make it plain. What does this mean for me?"

'When you go through deep waters and great trouble, I will be with you. When you go through rivers of difficulty, you will not drown. When you walk through the fire of oppression, you will not be burned up – the flames will not consume you. For I am the Lord your God, your Savior, the Holy One of Israel.'

It is a comfort God promises to be with me in this coming struggle – whatever it is. I see my part is to trust him. But still, I don't like this warning of impending doom.

Will something happen to me personally or to someone in my congregation? Not to my beloved son, oh God, please. Not to Jacob or his bride, Jessie. Please, God. I can't stand it.

Deep water and great trouble. Rivers of difficulty and the fire of oppression. And no hope that it might not happen because you preface everything with the word, "When."

When you go through it. When it happens. Three times I see a "When." Yet I do not understand.

Oh God, my God, I do trust you will be with me – no matter what happens. If it is an illness or a tragedy of some kind, you will not leave me to go through it alone. You are indeed the Lord my God, my Savior, my Comforter, my eternal Husband and Maker.

Help me to be brave. And help me to face whatever it is with my faith intact. Let me never, ever falter. Amen and Amen.

Like Reverend G during this season of change, I wonder about my mother's soul thoughts. How does she approach the shadows on her plastic blinds in assisted living? Does she remember the changing colors of the trees on the farm? Does she long for those autumnal moments or have they completely retreated in the Alzheimer-forming plaque that captures her brain?

I so want her to remember this season of autumn for its beauty, the crisp air and the promise of harvest. I long for my mother to recall with joy the way we celebrated with church folks, placed our foods in proper places for the giant potluck and sang, "We Gather Together to Ask the Lord's Blessing."

I hope Mom rejoices still in that sacred holy of holies inside her soul, that she somehow catches a tune from the past, the aroma of pumpkin pies cooling on the cabinet and the presence of her beloved Hank next to her.

And just in case my genes fail me and throw me also into Alzheimer's shadows, I will rejoice in the now. While I can, I will enjoy today. I will continue to walk in the crisp air, crunch tiny acorns under my feet and praise God for the colors and textures of autumn.

For how can we deal with shadows but to look for the remaining light? And how can we face something as horrific as Alzheimer's unless we gaze beyond it to the harvest of heaven?

LIVING THROUGH THE SEVEN STAGES

What are the stages of Alzheimer's Disease and how do they manifest in our loved ones?

Various scientific researchers will list the stages according to regression or lack of development, but I approach the question from the viewpoint of the caregiver and from our family's experience with Mom.

Stage 1: Preparation

No cognitive decline was present, but Mom sensed something was wrong. She didn't feel normal and wondered what was going to happen to her. She believed God might be preparing her for something in the near future, but she was going to fight against it. She constantly prayed, "Please, God. Don't let me get Alzheimer's."

Although many of us may forget why we're standing in front of the refrigerator or what we came into the room to find, Mom began to experience this phenomenon more often. Especially as a nurse, she believed it to be more than the natural aging process or the result of stress.

For caregivers, listen to your loved one. If they express concern, be alert for small changes and try to encourage them. At this point, no one knows the exact diagnosis and we need to live in joy as long as possible.

Stage 2: Questions

The seemingly insignificant symptoms of forgetfulness may become more frequent, but nothing impairs life. One example from Reverend G is how she forgets a line from "The Lord's Prayer."

A trip to the grocery store became troubling for Mom. She lost her grocery list and forgot everything she had written on it. She misplaced keys or her purse and was concerned she may have lost money in her checking account. Any issues surrounding money caused anxiety.

At this stage, caregivers may consider allergy testing, the effects of stress or the side effects of some medicines. For women, urinary tract infections can lead to confusion. Be wise, but don't give up yet. It may not be Alzheimer's after all.

Stage 3: Fear

Something was definitely wrong and life became more difficult. Confusion became a regular companion and the regular routines changed. Mom forgot where she kept the pots and pans. She still drove her car, but always parked in the same area at the grocery store so she could find it. She learned coping skills and for many months, we didn't notice the changes. She safety pinned her house keys to her slacks so she wouldn't lose them.

Her constant fear revolved around money. She was always asking, "Where is my purse?" – even when it was right in front of her. We began to see more anger which was probably connected to the fear. She repeated questions more often and short-term memory began to fade.

Caregivers often begin to deny what is happening. They, too, pick up on the fear and possibly the anger. Patience is necessary when the same questions are asked over and over. It's time to consider some medical answers, but caregivers will have to make the appointment and become the advocate for their loved ones.

Our mother was NEVER going to admit she might have Alzheimer's and the last place she wanted to go was the doctor's office. She would also NEVER admit to the fear, but I could feel it surrounding her.

Stage 4: Diagnosis

The actual diagnosis of Alzheimer's often comes after death when the brain can be autopsied and studied, but with Mom – we had a firm diagnosis from an MRI. She also suffered from a type of brain cyst that was not malignant but could not be removed.

As I researched for the Reverend G books and also to help Mom any way possible, I discovered Type A personalities – like my mother – are more prone to dementia and Alzheimer's. The stresses of perfectionism, of extreme productivity and of constantly wearing out the brain with thought processes began to take their toll.

This is why it is so important to set healthy boundaries around our time, take a true Sabbath rest and learn how to enjoy life with more relaxing and fun activities.

For Mom, short-term memory claimed its possession in brain fog although her long-term memory seemed intact. She remembered activities and people from long ago, but forgot what she ate for breakfast that day. In fact, we began to notice how many days she forgot to eat.

For caregivers, know your loved one well. We did NOT tell Mom about the diagnosis because we knew it would only bring added stress and discouragement. We began to consider what types of assisted living facilities might be available, and my siblings started working on power of attorney paperwork.

Stage 5: Early Dementia

Mom no longer cared about time or the days of the week. She had difficulty counting backwards although she still knew our names, especially the grandchildren. Making decisions was difficult, so if we took her out to eat – we had to help her order a meal.

Her dreams seemed so real, she believed they actually happened so nightmares were particularly disturbing. She believed people were stealing her clothes, stealing her money and often – we were the enemy. It was a hard time for all of us, but we understood Mom wasn't really herself and she was dealing with life from the regression of an adolescent.

Caregivers will need additional patience during this stage and a proactive plan for caring for their loved one. This is a good time to get connected with a support group and determine how each of you will be involved in visiting your loved one and/or making decisions. It is also important to deal with family dynamics as they arise so siblings aren't pitted against each other and the surviving spouse doesn't feel left out.

Stage 6: Back to Childhood

Severe cognitive decline now becomes the prognosis. Expressive aphasia may be added to the mix as speech becomes more difficult and the meanings of words forgotten. Think back to when your children were learning to talk. The same thing is happening now, except in reverse and it isn't cute anymore.

Mom was now in assisted living and completely dependent on others for her survival. She forgot major events and the evening news meant nothing to her. She didn't care about the presidential election of 2016 or the increased incidents of earthquakes in

Oklahoma. She followed the rules at assisted living, but could no longer play Bingo or card games because comprehension was affected. Sometimes she acted like a rebellious child and refused to eat. The seasons of the year meant nothing as time virtually disappeared. Grooming became an issue.

Her faith, however, remained strong as she read her Bible every day. She could not tell us what she read, and we would often find her sitting in the dark with her Bible on her lap. I wondered if she saw Jesus or if angels came to comfort her.

For the caregiver, enjoy every moment your loved one still knows you. That joy may soon disappear as the next stage of Alzheimer's represents the end of all verbal communication.

Stage 7: The Race is Won

In this final stage, Alzheimer's patients are virtually infants. All speech is gone. Feeding and toileting need assistance. They lose the ability to walk and are bedridden. Unless God takes them to heaven, they will require moving into the final memory care units. Medicines may help them sleep or keep them from constant agitation. This is a good time to begin looking into the services of Hospice.

Although it is sad to reach this stage, we can still live in hope. We don't know exactly what our loved ones hear or perceive. We don't know what thoughts they may have, so it is important to continue to touch them, pray with them, encourage them and sing to them.

Music resides in the part of the brain that disappears last, so we can often communicate with old hymns or a familiar song. The presence of children and/or pets may still bring comfort but we often won't know because our loved ones can't communicate with us. They are basically infants within adult bodies.

Caregivers may begin to plan for final arrangements. Don't wait to make all the final decisions when grief overwhelms. Hopefully, your loved one has already communicated her wishes to you. Our mother – always the planner – had everything ready and paid for long before she experienced even the first symptoms.

Remember to take care of yourself during each of these stages. This journey is a marathon and you may be involved for ten years or more.

In the end, as shown in "Final Grace for Reverend G," even a fictional character can help us understand once we belong to God – he will never, ever let us go.

CALLING MOM

We used to chat for at least 30 minutes about recipes, her grandchildren or my latest writing project. She asked me about life in Kansas, and I listened to her descriptions of the weather and activities in Oklahoma.

We discussed the weather because it affected the various crops. She knew farm life still flowed through my veins. I missed the country. She knew without my telling her.

But now, with Alzheimer's stealing her brain cells, Mom cannot initiate phone conversations. She can answer basic yes and no questions, but she cannot reason her way through open-ended questions. She cannot tell me about new recipes or express interest in my writing projects. She remembers her grandson's name and always asks about him, but our conversations rarely last longer than five minutes.

I make a list of things to talk about, because she will not and cannot introduce new topics.

"How are you today, Mom?"

"Okay."

"Have you had any rain this week?"

"No."

"Is the food still good?"

"Yes. Good food."

Then I pause to swallow my tears and try to think of some way to initiate a longer answer— anything to hear more of her personality come through, that sense of humor we once shared or maybe a nugget about her faith.

"What do you think, Mom, about the election?"

"Oh. Hmm." She hands the phone back to my sister. She is obviously tired of talking and she has run out of answers.

Although it is difficult to talk to Mom now and carry on any type of relevant chat, I still call every week. Because I need to hear her voice.

I know someday even that will be gone.

If your parents are still living, call them often. Call today. Initiate a conversation and take the time to call – while you can, while someone still answers.

KEEPING MOM BUSY

One of the rites of passage as teenagers was to choose activities we enjoyed and find others that strengthened our natural giftings. Some of these activities led us to pursue life-long interests and even helped us choose college majors or careers.

What I did not realize until I became a parent was the importance of activities to keep kids involved and out of trouble. It is important to keep our children busy while still allowing them some time to rest and play.

Now I see the importance of activities for my elderly mother. The activities' director at Mom's assisted living facility is always busy coordinating fun things for the residents. Most of these activities are not only enjoyable but also a bit mentally challenging – which is a good way to stave off the effects of Alzheimer's.

During the Christmas season, Mom and her friends ride the shuttle to see the lights and watch the local Christmas pageant. In the summer, they board the shuttle to attend Cowboy Church where they sing Country Western hymns and listen to the pastor talk about freedom in Jesus – with his appropriate Wrangler jeans and silver belt buckle.

Back at the facility, Mom plays cards every day, sometimes three times a day. Usually Uno or Skipbo. They don't keep score because who cares?

Other activities include a Bible study called Devotions with Doughnuts, weekly salon appointments and the walk around the pond or watching fish swim in the aquarium.

Once a week, residents gather for Bingo which reminds me of Roxie, the activities director for Reverend G, who calls out the numbers so Chris, Bert or Reverend G can win.

Mom often wins a Snickers bar or sometimes a little posey for her apartment. When I visit, she opens her drawer full of Snickers and gives them to me. "Take these back to Caleb," she says. "He likes them."

My son doesn't really care about candy that much, but he'll take anything from his grandma. She seems happy to give something away, so that's what counts.

We're glad Mom is so busy enjoying these activities, but it is becoming more difficult for my siblings and I to visit her. We have to schedule our visits between Bingo, doughnuts and the ever-present Uno game.

I'm glad Mom is busy. It keeps her out of trouble.

NECKS VERSUS BRAINS

A few weeks ago, I read Nora Ephron's memoir about aging: "I Feel Bad About My Neck." With her usual wit and masterful use of the English language, Nora wrote honestly about her own aging issues.

She included essays about the neck and how it quickly turns from smooth, soft skin into something resembling a turkey wattle. Also included were humorous details about how we disguise age with hair dye, moustache bleach and various versions of face lifts and Botox.

I laughed at Nora's descriptions and agreed with her assumptions that at some point, no one cares how old we are or how well we disguise it.

But I wondered if Nora wanted to include some essays about the aging of the brain and how that worry surpasses all the physical symptoms of living beyond 50.

Did she ever experience the sudden lapse of a long-remembered name when she could picture the face of a childhood friend but could not for the life of her – recall the name belonging to the face?

Did Nora ever make frequent visits to her file cabinet to look up something she had just looked up five minutes ago?

Did this talented writer and long-time journalist ever forget a word and wonder where her brain catalogued it?

Did Nora fear words, phrases and sentences might someday become lost within the aging plaque of her brain – thus deleting her writing career?

Maybe writing about brain aging was a little too scary, too painfully honest to include in her book. Or perhaps Nora remained gratefully alert even in her dying moments, God rest her soul.

But she did indicate a slight worry when she wrote, "Is life too short or is it going to be too long?"

Nora's book provided a humorous recess between my visits to Mom in assisted living and celebrating the holidays with my Oklahoma family.

But with Alzheimer's attacking my mother's brain and dementia pulsing through my father's genes, the aging I worry about is much scarier than grey hair or wrinkles.

With the dangers of brain atrophy and what that might involve, I will be grateful if the only part of me that ages is my neck.

FORGETTING MOM

I worked at my day job 10 hours, rushed home to water the flowers before they bent their sad little heads and shriveled up, exercised a bit, ate a few bites – then sat down at the computer to write, fell into bed and did it all over again the next day.

But with all the busy-ness of my week, something worse happened. I forgot Mom.

Each week, I send her a card. Usually, I shop at Dollar Tree where cards are only 50 cents, fun cards with little animals or happy faces – usually in the kid's section.

Then I go home and write a little something to Mom about my work or about her grandson. I pray over the card, ask God to help my mother through another day of Alzheimer's and stamp it for mailing the next day.

As the long distance caregiver in the family, this is my weekly attempt to assuage the almost daily guilt I feel because I cannot be there for Mom. I send a card and hope somehow through the miles, she will hear my love and know how sorry I am I cannot do more.

But this week – with all the extra activities and craziness – I forgot to send the card.

I romped along in my busy life, helped several women with their issues, coached my clients, wrote a blog post, spoke at a church event, worked on my novel – and totally forgot about Mom's card.

Guilt sandwiched between two slabs of more guilt.

On one side of my heart, I know it doesn't matter. Mom never remembers when I send cards and sometimes – even with my signature scrawled on the bottom – she tells people my cards came from her sister.

But even if she can't remember, I need her to receive my cards and to believe that I care. I need it because even if she doesn't care about the cards, I do.

I know I need to deal with the guilt and one of these days, when life is not so crazy – I will grieve my way through it and write pages in my journal or enough blog posts and books to somehow bandage the grief.

In the meantime, I'll send another card – right now – and hope Mom will open it in a couple of days, laugh at the kitty on the front and tell somebody, "This is from my daughter in Kansas."

ALZHEIMER'S AT THE WEDDING

Throughout the pre-wedding activities for my niece and her beau, Mom functioned well. She attended bridal showers, listened to all the exciting plans and smiled for the photographer.

But we knew our 85 year-old mother might create a few problems on the actual wedding day. It was my job to get Mom dressed, drive her to the church and make sure she made it down the aisle.

I was surprised at the changes in Mom. From the last time I saw her in May until the wedding date in July, she had regressed further into the disease. Her facial expressions resembled those of a child, that naughty rolling-the-eyes look. When we discussed what she would wear to the wedding, I had to go through the scenario several times.

"We talked about this skirt, Mom. It's a nice skirt."

"No, I want to wear the red one."

"Not a good choice of color, Mom. Red is too dark for a summer wedding and besides, it has a spot on the front. Did you tell them to launder it?"

"Yes." A debatable answer, because Mom's short-term memory grows shorter every week.

Finally, she pulled on a turquoise skirt, and I convinced her to wear a beautiful white blouse with a lacy collar. As I fluffed up her hair, I asked, "Don't you have some pretty pearl earrings? They would look nice."

"No. All my jewelry has been stolen." Paranoia is strong these days. Mom is convinced everyone in the facility and her own family members have stolen her jewelry, her money, even her clothes.

When she was finally dressed, I drove us to the church. But pictures were scheduled for noon and the wedding for two o'clock. Two hours is a long time for someone whose concept of time has disappeared.

First, we ate lunch – slowly. I tried to convince Mom to eat more meat and drink more water, but she refused. However, she sat quietly and waited while I finished eating. My brother came to escort her for some of the outdoor pictures, then brought her back to me.

Mom and I strolled through the church and looked at the beautiful decorations. Lanterns along the sides of the pews. Purple and green petals strewn up and down the aisle. Beautiful cascades of dark purple gladiola at the front of the sanctuary. Everything ready for that moment when our Rachel would walk down the aisle to meet her love, Grant.

Surely Mom would remember these precious moments. "How about if we tour the library, Mom? Would you like to see the church library?"

"Oh, yes. I like books."

So we toured the library, picked out a few to look at and discussed others. "They have a good selection here," I said.

"Yes," Mom said. "I like books."

I remembered when she helped organize and catalog our church library. I also remembered when a prayer group met in the library, and my mother was one of the members — a praying woman who cared about overseas missions. Mom not only prayed for missionaries, but she also gave a portion of her nursing salary to help meet those same missionaries' needs.

That was a long time ago — before Alzheimer's stole Mom's ability to help in a church library or participate in a prayer group.

In a few minutes, Mom tired of the library so we walked through the church again. We watched the photographer shoot pictures of Rachel and Grant. Then Mom grew restless.

"Hey, Mom. Would you like to go see the church library?"

"Oh, yes. I like books."

Three times we toured the library, each time about twenty minutes apart. Then we sat in the fellowship hall and watched people file into the sanctuary. The wedding planner found us and fastened a flowered bracelet on Mom wrist.

"Why do I have to wear this?" she asked me. "You don't have one."

"Because you're special. You're the only grandparent on both sides of the families. You get to have a special flower."

"Well, okay," she said. Then about two minutes later, "Why do I have to wear this thing?"

Her grandson, Ethan came and held out his arm to escort her down the aisle. But Mom balked. "I don't want to do that. Everybody will be looking at me."

"No, Mom. They'll be waiting for Rachel. They want to see the bride. You just walk in quietly with Ethan."

"But if it's just Ethan and me, then they'll be looking at me and I look fat in this skirt. I shouldn't have worn this skirt. I should have a nicer outfit."

"Now, Mom. This is Rachel's special day. Ethan will take care of you, so you just walk down the aisle with him and then sit by me at the front. Remember, this is for Rachel."

Mom rolled her eyes. I fully expected her to stick out her tongue, but after another grimace, she took Ethan's arm. I joined my son, my sister, my aunt and her daughter in the second row and watched as Ethan and Mom came down the aisle.

Even within the horror of Alzheimer's disease, Mom was a trooper. She paraded down the aisle and smiled while doing it. She did her part for her granddaughter's special day. Rachel married Grant and Mom lived through it.

I was proud of her and also relieved. We made it through two hours of waiting and Mom's few minutes in the spotlight. Even within the shadows of Alzheimer's, we found some joy.

LONG-DISTANCE CAREGIVING

A friend recently encouraged me to define my role as a long-distance caregiver. At first, I wondered how this defined role might help me deal with the guilt and anxiety I feel whenever I drive away from Mom.

But the more I thought about it, the more I liked the idea. Define my role and maybe even give myself a job description to help deal with this nasty Alzheimer's diagnosis that consumes our family.

Certainly, those who care full-time for Alzheimer's and/or dementia patients have the greatest stress. It is rightly described as the 36-hour day. Yet each person in the family is affected in some way by this horrific disease that takes away our loved ones piece by fractured piece.

As the LDC in my family, I live 250 miles away from Mom. The rest of my family lives in the same area, our wonderful and cozy home town of Enid, Oklahoma.

For years, I have driven I-35 South on major holidays and whenever I could pull away from ministry here in Kansas. Now that Mom lives in assisted living, I still try to observe holidays and any other important family events. But I cannot be there all the time. Thus, the necessity of my title – the LDC, long-distance caregiver.

What then is my job description? How can I best encourage my siblings and support them from a distance? How can I help Mom or is that beyond possibility?

I believe my job description includes five topics:

Keep in Regular Contact

I try to call my sister each week and my brother each month. We talk about different things: sports, the weather and how it will affect this year's wheat crop, the activities of nieces and nephews. Then we talk about Mom.

"How's she doing this week? Does she seem more content with her new living situation? Any changes? Any problems?"

Asking questions and hearing the answers helps me feel a bit more connected to what is happening in this process. Plus, it gives me ideas for how to pray—not only for Mom but also for my siblings.

Sometimes I hear the frustration in their voices. Sometimes I catch a bit of the anger and grief we all feel because our mother has this disease. Often I want to hug my siblings through the cell phone towers and let them know how much I care for them, how much I miss them.

Ultimately, the LDC in me has to depend on God and his promise in Psalm 54:4, "Surely God is my help; the Lord is the one who sustains me."

Research for New Helps

Since I am an author and write about finding hope when life unravels, I study everything I can find about caregiving, Alzheimers and how families can help their loved ones. Sometimes I come up with a new coping strategy. Sometimes, my siblings already know more than I do.

Recently, I discovered information about urinary tract infections. Apparently, older women can easily contract UTIs, yet don't always feel the pain.

They cannot tell us how or where it hurts. Yet one of the symptoms of a UTI is frightening and realistic nightmares.

My mother has nightmares that seem so real to her, she reports them to the staff at the assisted living facility. She is certain various family members are stealing her car, her money or her house because she has dreamed these scenarios in living color.

Mom concocts the most amazing stories, based on her dreams. She could have been an incredible novelist. Her stories are fascinating and believable.

More than once, the staff has called my sister to check up on one of Mom's stories. When I told my sister about the research on UTIs, she scheduled a doctor appointment to have Mom checked.

Mom's stories are one of the side effects of Alzheimer's or maybe even some of the medicines she takes. But now that we know about UTIs, we can be more alert for a possible cause for future stories.

Even though I cannot always find answers to the questions we have, doing the research helps me feel as if I have an active part in Mom's care. As the LDC and the researcher, I am doing something beneficial and helping the family take care of Mom.

I am also learning more about this disease and trying to prevent it from happening to me. I eat a Mediterranean diet, try to avoid anything cooked or stored in aluminum, and I've completely eliminated high fructose corn syrup from my diet.

Beyond that, I plead with God every day to help my siblings as they care for Mom and keep us all from getting this horrid disease.

Be Observant About the Changes

As Mom slips away with each visit, I see the changes. Sometimes I am more aware of these changes than my siblings because they see her all the time.

I notice Mom's drawn face, her added confusion, the fear that has always plagued her – now increasing. I share these observations with my siblings and we try to make the important decisions necessary to help Mom through each stage.

The delicate balance is that I cannot just breeze into town, tell everybody what I have observed and expect them to listen to my incredible advice.

Just because I'm the oldest doesn't mean I'm the smartest or the most discerning. It just means I'm the oldest. Darn it!

But even one of my relatives once told me, "I'll bet you can see the changes easier than we can."

Yes, that's true. During the Easter holiday, I noticed how withdrawn Mom had become. Was it because her hearing aid needed adjusting or had she lost more comprehension? Was she not able to understand conversation as easily as she did at Christmas? A few months can make a world of difference to an Alzheimer's victim.

Mom and I share some of the some personality traits. We're both choleric, Type A's—those get- busy-and-get-it-done women who organize the world while telling everyone what to do and how to do it.

My life experiences and my training as a life coach and a Stephen minister have taught me to temper my choleric self, to listen carefully and help people see the solutions themselves.

So even though I might see the changes, I cannot march in and suggest a solution. No answers exist for Alzheimer's. All we can do is persevere through each 36-hour day, hang on to our faith and pray for everyone involved.

Together, my siblings and I make an awesome team. My sister is smart, and my brother is wise. I add the fresh eyes to observe Mom's changes.

As a family, we blend our love for Mom and our life experiences into the best caregiving unit we can possibly be.

Still, observing the changes in Mom also helps me see the changes in all of us as we age, deal with the stress of caregiving and search every resource for the best way to make it through this journey.

May God help us so even as we observe the changes, we will also learn grace to accept them.

Be Alert for Emotional Dynamics

Living with Alzheimer's and/or dementia causes a host of emotions—especially for caregivers.

Mom's emotions aren't that difficult. She lives in a contented land where all she has to worry about is where she put her teeth during the night and can she find her underwear the next day. Even then, somebody helps her with those problems.

But for the rest of us, it's a different story. Until I entered this journey with my siblings, I had no idea of the emotions that would swirl around us.

As the LDC, there is of course, the emotion of guilt. But it is a false guilt, a self-condemnation because I cannot be in Oklahoma all the time, helping with Mom.

At the same time, I am grateful for my life in Kansas and the work I do. I am proud of the ministry and the incredible women I help as well as my growing coaching practice and my writing life.

Guilt raises its ugly head whenever something happens, and I am too far away to help. Then when I visit Mom, guilt rides home with me because I can drive away and my siblings cannot.

Another emotion with tremendous affect is grief. One possible advantage of dealing with Alzheimer's is that we grieve little by little rather than in one traumatic explosion. With each change and every increase in confusion, with each memory lapse, we grieve a little more. We understand these lapses will grow in frequency until Mom no longer knows who we are.

We also know someday, Mom will stop breathing and this horrid journey will be over. So we will not have to deal with the terrible shock of a tragic death. Mom is dying a little bit every day, right in front of us.

As the LDC, I grieve for the stress this disease adds to my siblings and to all our family. Some of us express anger while others struggle with health problems as a result of the stress.

Each time I drive to Oklahoma and then back to Kansas, it takes about 10 days to process my emotions, journal through them and return to some place of normalcy. I can only imagine the emotional toll on my siblings.

These emotions may never ease until the very end of Mom's journey. In the meantime, we will grow our need for more grace.

This is why it is important for caregivers to take care of ourselves – whether we're right in the thick of it or dealing with it long distance.

Emotions can tear us apart or make us stronger. I hope to finish well.

Pray

My personal intercessory team lifts me up in prayer before every trip to Oklahoma, my return trips to Kansas and everything in between.

My siblings also have people in their churches, their cell groups and their networks who pray for them.

Certainly, we all pray for Mom. I pray she will not have to suffer long. I am begging God to take her home where she can be with Jesus, with Dad and with her parents.

What is the point of pretending? Mom is a strong believer. Her faith is intact even if her brain is scrambled. I pray God will release her soon so she can go home.

Every night and sometimes during the daytime hours, I pray for my sister. I have seen how her health has been affected. Stress wreaks havoc on our bodies, so I pray for my sister to find relief from the pain, to sleep well and to find the joy of living.

I pray for my brother as he juggles work on the farm along with his other job, his family and the dynamics all of that brings. I pray for him special grace because he works hard, and I ask God to bless him in many ways.

Then I pray for me, that as I live through this long distance caregiving experience, I will approach my role with grace.

In the end, Alzheimer's does not win. What really counts is how we deal with our family dynamics and how we stay close to each other – even when we live far apart.

What matters is how we share what we have learned. Because that is why we are here: to love God, to make a difference and to leave well.

Part of that leaving well is a legacy of wisdom and experience for those who come behind us. To let them know that even in the journey of Alzheimer's, prayer is still the best thing we can do.

In the end, our role is to enjoy our loved ones as long as possible and not kill ourselves in the process. We know caregiving is stressful, but if we do it right – we can be a blessing to each other and make it through this unraveling journey.

LIVING IN THE SATURDAYS

A pocket of time separates Good Friday and Easter Sunday – a day we often ignore. We don't celebrate the Saturday between – we just wait.

We live through Saturday, anticipating Sunday.

After the execution of Jesus, the disciples huddled together in fear. At least one of them, Peter, hid alone, ashamed of his refusal to acknowledge he was a follower of Jesus.

This band of scared and incredibly human disciples waited during Saturday, daring to hope, wondering what Sunday might bring. Surely they waited for a knock on the door, for angry soldiers to arrest them and sentence them to the same treatment their Master had suffered.

Waiting. Dreading. Vascillating between hope and despair.

Hadn't he said something about rising from the dead? Did he mean that literally?

We are often stuck in the same time warp.

During the Fourth of July weekend in 2008 , my son was diagnosed with a brain tumor. Fireworks. Patriotic songs. The joy of a national holiday.

Yet in one tragic moment, an astrocytoma's ferocious prognosis changed our lives. Surgery. Chemotherapy. Radiation. A treatment plan that included years of MRI's, oncologist appointments and escalating medical bills.

A lifetime of Saturdays, waiting, hoping, praying. Then the glorious ending five years later – a miraculous healing with no recurrence. Our resurrection Sunday arrived with joy.

But the Saturdays required guts and perseverance.

My mother stepped into the shadows of Alzheimers. Thousands and thousands of Saturdays morphed into 36-hour days as she changed from a mature and intelligent woman into a child-like version of herself.

Day follows day and years repeat until one day, the waiting ends. On that day, we will lower her shell into the ground. She knows this. We anticipate and dread it, while knowing that moment will signify her release from this travesty.

The crosses of our lives thrust us into expanded weekends as we experience pain, separation and the perseverance of waiting.

We know on some level the pain does end. Resurrection follows crucifixion.

But it is the waiting during our Saturdays that threatens to shove us into discouragement. Saturdays seem interminable as we beg God to send us Easter sunrise.

Yet within our Saturdays, as character is tested and perseverance questioned, we learn eternal lessons about faith.

Hope that endures requires massive faith and teeth-grinding strength for the length of the journey.

Because we must wait through the Saturdays, the end result seems that much sweeter when Easter Sunday finally arrives.

BIRTHDAY CHANGES

All my life, Mom made my birthday a special event. One year, she made the most decadent gooey chocolate cake I have ever tasted. I walked into the house after a long basketball practice, plopped into my chair at the kitchen table and eagerly sliced a piece of that wonderful cake.

It tasted like love.

During my first year of college, I lived in the far away land of Arkansas. But on my birthday, Mom somehow managed to send a message to the dorm mother who arranged for a chocolate chip creation I shared with all the girls on my hall.

Mom never forgot birthdays for any of us. She planned for weeks to bake the best cake, find the perfect present and make the day special. Then she lustily sang the Happy Birthday song, to ensure that each of her children knew what a special day it was for her, too.

During the years of our Alzheimer's journey, my birthdays taste bittersweet. One year on my birthday, I signed books in my hometown Hastings. It was a great time of connecting with friends and family, talking about Reverend G and sipping an iced chai. Afterwards, my siblings and I feasted at the local Western Sizzlin' where I treated myself to a dish of blackberry cobbler a la mode.

Then I drove to the nursing home to spend the rest of the evening with Mom. We watched television together and she asked me over and over about my son's major in college. I didn't tell her about the book signing, because she would have regretted that she couldn't come.

Every five minutes, she pleaded, "When can I go home? Why can't I go home? I want to go home."

No birthday card. No mention of the day. No gooey chocolate chip cake.

I felt guilty for my self-pity, knowing that for me it was only a birthday. For Mom, my special day only represented a moment in the rest of her life, dwelling in a facility and the gradual eating away of her brain by the brutal Alzheimer's Disease.

But still, I miss the fact that October 12th now passes without a birthday acknowledgement from Mom. No more decadent chocolate chip cakes, no colorful balloons, no Happy Birthday song. Those days are finished.

Instead, I cling to the memories of birthdays past and hang on to the only One who never changes, the Christ who saved me and upholds all of us in this Alzheimer's journey with Mom.

ALMOST LYING

A TV pastor recently said, "White lies don't exist. A lie is a lie, and deception is always wrong. Tell the whole truth."

While I understood what he was trying to teach, I wondered if he had any loved ones struggling through Alzheimer's Disease?

One of the issues my siblings and I now face is that we sometimes we have to tell Mom an almost-lie. It feels like deception and in the black and white world of that TV preacher, it probably is.

But the entire truth sounds like a cruel answer to a simple question. For example, every day and many times a day, Mom asks, "When can I go home?"

The absolute truth is, "You're not going home, Mom – not today, not ever. You're going to stay here in assisted living until Alzheimer's steals the rest of your brain and you end up in the nursing home section of this facility. The next stop after that is the cemetery, but your spirit will be in heaven with Dad and Jesus, so you won't care."

The almost-lie is, "Maybe in two weeks you can go home, Mom, depending on what the doctor says." Then after two weeks, the answer is still, "Maybe in two weeks." And two weeks after that...ditto.

Thus, two weeks becomes a month which becomes 12 months and a year, which is the scenario for the Alzheimer's patient.

We have learned the kindest way to respond to Mom is to tell her the same almost-lie every day. Since time and space have disappeared, she accepts these answers and seems more peaceful.

Contentment resides within the almost-lie.

Helping Mom through this stage of her disease means not telling her the entire brutal truth, but trying to create a temporary world she can somehow accept.

But inside my gut, it still feels like a a terrible transgression and the breaking of the ninth commandment.

With Alzheimer's, the borders of the black and white box fade. Right versus wrong needs to be reconfigured. Grey is also a color and for now, the grey world is where we live.

In eternity, the truth will finally reveal itself. Then we will stand on the hope that both God and Mom will forgive us.

ART BECOMES LIFE

Oscar Wilde opined how life often imitates art, but once in a while, the philosophy reverses as art *becomes* life. I've seen it happen with my Reverend G series.

In "Final Grace for Reverend G," the main character purchases birthday cards for her son, Jacob, long before she begins to recede into the shadows of Alzheimer's. She wants to celebrate his day and encourage him even when she no longer remembers his birth date.

When my son celebrated his 29th birthday, he opened an interesting card from his grandmother. Although Mom hasn't read any of the Reverend G books nor have I told her what Reverend G does in "Final Grace," art became life.

My sister found a birthday card Mom purchased several years ago. It was already signed with Caleb's name on the envelope. In Mom's tiny scrawl were the same words she always used for his birthday cards, "Love you bunches – Grandma Arlene."

Did she have some sort of premonition that this one card would be sent when she no longer remembered dates, when time itself became an extinct commodity in her mind?

Did she hope her first grandchild would still cherish the grandmother who sits in assisted living and makes up stories she believes are true?

Did she want him to know although she cannot remember his age or his career, she cares enough to ask the same questions over and over, "How's Caleb? Is he doing okay? Tell him I think about him all the time."

Did she wonder if she would still be living when that card was delivered? Or would it be the last greeting she would send to this boy she loved?

When art becomes life, it gives me pause as a writer. Because I pray before I write and dedicate my words to the One who is the Word, I wonder how much of what pours out of me will manifest in the future.

Writers use words for therapy and much of our past experiences show up in our books and characters. But we also face the responsibility of knowing the words we use today might actually become reality tomorrow.

It behooves those of us who write to be even more cautious and ever alert for the voice of the Word within.

May the words of my mouth and those of my pen be acceptable in Your sight, O Lord, my Savior and my God

THE ALZHEIMER'S SLUSH PILE

Is there a file somewhere that holds all the items Alzheimer's patients lose? Bobby pins, money, dishes, clothing, expensive hearing aids.

Sometimes those items are imagined lost, but even so – the person struggling with Alzheimer's is convinced the object exists yet has simply disappeared. Where did it go?

My mother has lost a seersucker pantsuit. As far as I know, she never bought a seersucker pantsuit although she always wanted one. However, this suit is so real to her, it must exist somewhere in the universe, if not hanging in her closet. Perhaps she once bought one, but now – it has disappeared.

Where did it go? Does it wait in an imaginary pile hidden from the world of reality?

We no longer take jewelry to Mom, because it *will* disappear. Then Mom will accuse someone of stealing it. And truthfully, when Mom loses something, it cannot be found.

Jewelry *has* disappeared as well as the infamous seersucker pantsuit. How do you lose a pantsuit? Seersucker or any other variety? This puzzles me.

We no longer take Mom's hearing aids to her room, because lost hearing aids cost a bundle to replace. So my sister has become the Guardian of the Hearing Aids, producing them only when Mom goes to church or joins us for a family outing.

The rest of the time, Mom just doesn't hear well. She turns up the volume on her TV and when someone talks to her, she asks, "How's that? What? Huh?"

Mom has lost socks – but then, who hasn't lost a sock. They constantly run away from home.

Mom has lost other pieces of clothing and important documents. We know better than to leave any legal papers with Mom.

Yet she never loses cards. Her collection of greeting cards sent by friends and family sit in a basket, waiting for her to reread them. So far, she has not lost the basket or any of the cards.

Because Mom is always giving things away, she sometimes thinks she has lost something when she actually gave it away. She often wins at Bingo and wins Snickers candy bars. But she doesn't eat them. She gives them to grandkids, then doesn't remember giving them away. They hide in the Alzheimer's Slush File.

It doesn't really matter, I suppose, if Mom loses some things – as long as they aren't major items like hearing aids. The problem is that the disappearance of items causes Mom additional stress, and we don't know how to relieve that stress

Recently, I lost one of my favorite rings. I have no recollection of taking it off and putting it somewhere other than my jewelry case. I have looked in every suitcase, every container and every dresser drawer. My ring has disappeared. It only cost five dollars, but I liked it because it sparkled and matched lots of different outfits.

I have, of course, prayed, "Oh God, oh God, I have lost my ring. Please, please, please don't let me have Alzheimer's. Please let me find my ring."

He has not answered. I think my ring might be hiding with Mom's seersucker pantsuit.

WHEN DOUBT SWALLOWS FAITH

During a recent Bible study, we discussed the issue of doubt versus faith. I decided not to bother with the homework. After all, faith is one of my core values and also one of my spiritual gifts. I really have no problems with doubt.

Then I attended a networking meeting where a financial planner spoke. She provided sobering facts about the economy and our need to be prepared. One of the most chilling stats she quoted was the seventy per cent of Baby Boomers who will live in poverty during their retirement years.

As I listened to this bad news, I felt doubt and discouragement creep into my soul. I have tried to be careful and save money. Unfortunately, my savings account feels smaller every day.

So doubt crept in, replacing all my confident faith thoughts. What will I do if I face a major illness and cannot work? My financial plan is based on continuing to write and coach and work in ministry until God says, "You're done. Come home."

God has always provided for me. He often whispers, "I will take care of you."

But do I really believe that? Where is my faith?

Every time I visit my mother, I remind her how lucky she is. A woman who planned and saved throughout her lifetime, she also bought long-term care insurance when it was affordable. She now lives in a beautiful facility and all her needs are met. She never has to worry about bills.

I look around her beautiful room with all her comforts and a part of my soul envies her.

Even within the Alzheimer's journey, I envy Mom's cozy existence and wish I could hope for the same.

But where is my faith?

We may plan and save and hope for the best, but ultimately, none of us knows what life will hand us nor how long we will live.

Will life be short enough to utilize our careful plans or will it prove to be too long, leaving us in poverty when we cannot work our way out of it?

All I can do is be grateful Mom is comfortable while I keep working and doing what God tells me to do – keep believing God will indeed take care of me.

In the end, God is the best long-term insurance available.

MOM WALKS TALL

As a child, I thought my mother was literally ten feet tall. At 5'8", she towered over me both in height and in authority.

During the last few years, osteoporosis has reduced her spine. We are now the same height at 5'5". Now we gaze at each other on equal footing, although I still emotionally look up to her.

Lately, Mom has seemed taller again – or maybe she's just feistier.

For several months, she seemed content with her apartment in assisted living. "You're so lucky," I told her.

"This is such a beautiful place," Mom said. "I don't have to cook or clean here, and the food is good."

But during my recent visit, Mom regressed back to the anger she felt when we first moved her in as a resident. "I want to go home," she repeated. "I can't believe I'm here."

No amount of placating seemed to help. None of my comments about how lucky she is made a dent in her attitude. She had reverted back to anger and frustration, both of us ignoring the fact that Alzheimer's would keep her out of her home for the rest of her earthly life.

Yet her dogged determination persisted. She obeyed as my sister and I picked her up for church. "Put in your hearing aid, Mom. You'd better put on a sweater. It's cold outside. You'll need your scarf. It's windy."

But I could tell anger waited below the surface, along with

confusion and the strange reality that is now her life.

After a family lunch together, we drove Mom back to the assisted living facility. She stepped out of the car and let me hug her, but she wouldn't say, "I love you," even though I said it first.

I wanted so desperately to hear her say it. "I'm going back to Kansas," I reminded her. *Won't you please tell me you love me? Can't you forget the anger for a moment?*

Instead, she walked away with that perfect posture back into the facility – her shadow reflected on the windows as she proceeded down the hallway – back to her apartment, back to the place she doesn't want to be.

I don't want you there, either, and I don't want you to struggle with Alzheimer's.

I want to see her standing tall again over the kitchen sink or planting flowers in the garden or hanging wash on the line. My mother shouldn't be 85 years old with her complexion as white as her hair.

This is not fair, God. I can't stand it, and I'm sure Mom can't either.

I wonder…what does she do during the nighttime hours? Does she cry for the life she once had or has she forgotten it entirely?

Does she wonder how she came to live where she is now? Does she remember the confusion, how she passed out and needed a pacemaker? Does she realize the doctor told us she could no longer live alone?

Does she know how proud I am of her that she still walks tall?

SAGA OF THE TOWELS

Before we moved Mom to assisted living, I noticed her towels. Every towel in her house, kitchen and bathrooms was worn thin and bleached out. Drying off after a shower felt like rubbing sandpaper all over my body – great for exfoliation, not so great for comfort.

So I decided to update Mom's towels. I bought her a beautiful set, embroidered with a band of royal blue flowers. Blue – her favorite color and a bargain at K-Mart.

She loved the towels and promised to use them. I planned to buy another set for her birthday, then Mother's Day and Christmas – to gradually help her replace all the towels in the house.

But Alzheimer's set in, and Mom forgot where she put things. She started to hoard and hide. She gave away things she was supposed to keep and kept items that should have been trashed.

Her pots and pans? A daily search for the right cabinet. Her car registration form? In the bottom of the dumpster. The beautiful towels I gave her – a mystery.

When I visited, I asked her, "Where are the pretty blue towels? Haven't you been using them?"

"Oh, I don't know," she said.

We searched in all the logical places: the linen closet, the laundry, even the top of Mom's closet where she hides things she might someday use. No blue towels anywhere. I wondered if she gave them away or if they somehow landed in the trash can.

I wavered between anger at the loss of my gift and sadness for the disease that stole away so much of my mother's life, even the items she once loved.

What was the point of buying new towels for someone who forgot where she put them? Once again, I dried off with the same old sandpaper fabric.

Then we had to admit Mom to the assisted living facility where someone else took care of her laundry, including her towels. She seemed content. No worries and no memories.

But after she moved out of her house, it became easier to find the things she had buried in corners and crevices. Important papers resurfaced, suddenly alphabetized where they had previously lived in chaos. Fourteen boxes of SOS pads. I guess Mom bought them in case she needed to clean every cookie sheet in the state of Oklahoma. Lost socks that had previously decided to divorce their mates.

Then one weekend, I stayed with my sister in the family home. At bedtime, she came into the guest room and said, "Look what I found." She handed me a bundle of fuzzy comfort.

I hurried to the privacy of the bathroom, buried my face in the beautiful blue towels and grieved for another lost piece of my mother.

HIDING THE WORDS

During a recent hospital stay, Mom needed extra care and supervision. So to give my sister a break from the constant strain of caregiving, I opted to stay at the hospital with our mother.

One morning, Mom seemed especially agitated so I asked her, "What's your favorite Psalm?"

"Oh, probably 23," she said.

I pulled my Bible out of my purse and started reading from the English Standard Version.

Mom nodded her head, but then looked puzzled as I read, "Even though I walk through the valley of the shadow of death, I will fear no evil."

Mom peered at me from the sides of her trifocals and said, "I was thinking about the words while you read them. It should be 'Yea, though I walk through the valley.'"

"You're right, Mom. You learned it from the King James Version which says, 'Yea, though I walk.'"

Later, as she napped, I tried to smooth out the wrinkles in her hand. Such fragile skin. Almost no muscle or fat left on her entire body – this woman who made nutritious meals, exercised daily and carried herself with self-respect. This nurse who wore a cross necklace under her uniform to remind herself she belonged to Jesus.

Somewhere deeper than the shadows of Alzheimer's, entire

passages of the Bible lay cached in my mother's soul. Places where the beauty of the King James Version still lay, where a beloved Psalm was protected within the sacred compartment of divine memory.

Those verses we learn as children and repeat as adults stay with us. In the repository only God knows how to enter, the basics of our faith do not fail us – even when we forget our loved ones, even when we lose our language, even when we walk through the valley shadowed by death.

What a treasure to know my mother's faith stands firm, based on the Word of God which has not failed her and never will.

King David confirmed it in Psalm 119, "I have hidden your word in my heart."

Mom still believes it, still lives it, hiding God's word so deeply in her heart that nothing on earth can steal it away.

Not even Alzheimer's.

HOPE AT THE CAPITOL

To be chosen as one of the featured authors at the Kansas Book Festival seemed both a humbling and inspiring event.

Years ago, I toured the capitol building in Topeka and was impressed by its grandeur, the gold and bronze shining off light fixtures. The acoustics in the hallways. That rotunda with its dizzying majesty.

But this trip to the Capitol was different. I spoke in the Senate Chamber because my writing dream became reality.

As I shared with the audience about the Reverend G trilogy, I recognized despair in some of the faces. They knew in first person viewpoint what Alzheimer's Disease is all about.

Even from the podium, surrounded by plush leather chairs our senators sit in to make laws, I felt the need of my audience – their silent plea, *Please, help us make it through this journey.*

So I shared practical tips, told some funny stories – because we all need to laugh – and tried to let them know they were not alone.

After I spoke, several people came forward to meet me and shake my hand. One woman said, "I have a friend with Alzheimer's."

Another woman teared up as she said, "My husband has dementia."

A gentleman gushed, "Thank you for your encouragement."

Later, I met the other authors, companions in the art of crafting words. The author reception at Cedar Crest reminded me I am easily impressed. Give me a long table of hors d'oeuvres decorated with a beautiful spray of flowers and I am pleased. Let me walk through a spacious sunroom, complete with comfy chairs and Tiffany lamps and I am awe-struck. Sit me down in a library with a plateful of chocolate truffles and I am in earthly heaven.

To meet the governor and his wife – a privilege. To speak to the chef – a delight. To sign the Festival posters with the other authors – a pleasure.

But the most inspirational moment of the weekend came as I was leaving Cedar Crest. A panorama of trees formed an anchor for the setting sun. Off in the distance, a church steeple rose above the tree line, its cross pointing straight upward.

I stood for a moment in the cool of dusk and thanked God for the honor of sharing his words on the printed page. That he would call me to write and then allow me to be honored for what he had done seemed a strange irony. But then, God often encourages his children in radical ways.

He proves over and over that he is the one – the only one – who can make good happen in this mixed up world, even using the disease of Alzheimer's to somehow point us toward hope.

MOM'S UNCHANGING SMILE

One of her lifetime friends visited Mom in her apartment at assisted living. When Virginia entered the room, Mom looked up and smiled as if she remembered their years of service together, the sharing of Mennonite foods and the fellowship in a crowded sanctuary.

The smile remained fixed even as Mom's eyes registered surprise.

The three of us chatted about the weather. Mom repeated the same phrase several times, "So cold now. The ice...that's what you have to be careful of."

Virginia and I reminisced about another friend who had recently graduated to heaven. We talked about family and generations of connections, the folks who traveled long distances for the funeral, the nice service, the beautiful music.

Mom's smile remained in the same upturned pose. She seemed a world away.

Virginia asked about Mom's activities. "Do you like the food here?"

"Oh, yes. Wonderful food. I think I'm getting fat."

We all laughed. My slender mother has never struggled with her weight. Mom's smile widened. She seemed to enjoy the echoes of our laughter even though she may not have comprehended the humor.

A smile sometimes conveys a compliant spirit even while memory hides behind walls of dementia-covered plaque.

Then a break in the conversation – one of those lulls where no one knows what to say because every appropriate subject has been covered.

Mom filled in the gaps with the same statement as before. "The ice…you have to be careful of ice."

Virginia reached for her coat and found her gloves tucked into pockets. She hugged Mom good-bye, then hugged me. Her whisper touched my cheek with the slight smell of peppermint gum. "I'll pray for your mother, for all of you. Alzheimer's is such a terrible disease."

"Thank you. We appreciate that."

As she left, Mom's smile began to fade. Her eyes widened. "Who was that?" she asked.

"Your friend, Virginia. You used to be in the same Sunday School class. You went shopping together and met for coffee. She was a good friend."

"I see," said Mom, but her eyes registered no recollection.

Then she turned toward the winter-frosted window with a practiced smile.

HOPE RETURNS WITH A BOSSY MOM

I drove to Oklahoma to spend an afternoon with Mom. For the first time in months, she was fairly lucid, talking like her old self.

We took a walk around the perimeter of the facility, discussed the geese who flew onto the pond for a drink and goose fellowship.

Mom remarked how nice the facility was and how glad she was to live there – a reversal of the attitude she displayed during my last visit. "Why am I here? Why did you kids do this to me?"

Heartache piled upon guilt.

But on this day, she seemed grateful, and I saw in her the personality I grew up with – the bossy Mom who made sure her kids read at least seven books each week, practiced their musical instruments and completed their homework and chores.

Suddenly, we were transported decades before as Mom became herself.

"You need to hem up those pants you're wearing. They're dragging on the ground."

"I did hem them, Mom."

"Well, you need to do it again – another inch at least."

"Okay, Mom. When I get home."

Then we walked to the dining room. Mom instructed me where to sit. "Grab that chair over there. Someone else, a really old woman, always sits beside me. Show her respect and let her sit first."

"Okay, Mom. I'll do that."

As the meal was served, Mom wondered why I wasn't eating. "How come you don't have a plate? Do you want me to order one for you?"

"No. I stopped at Braum's two hours ago. I'm not hungry."

"Well, you'll be hungry by morning if you don't eat now. Do you want a cookie? I'll get you a cookie."

"No, thanks. I eat gluten free."

"Why?"

"Because I'm allergic to wheat."

Mom shook her head. "That can't be right. You grew up on a wheat farm and we had bread for every meal."

"Exactly why I'm probably allergic."

"Are you sure you don't want a cookie?"

The nurturing of children continues into old age, even when the brain is infected with Alzheimer's plaque. A mother longs to feed her children, to make sure they never go hungry, even if they are visiting, even if they have just eaten.

After Mom finished her meal, we walked back to her room. "Do you want to watch the idiot box?" (Mom's adjective for the TV).

"No. I'll just sit here with you and read my book."

"Yeah. There's nothing on but junk anyway."

We sat in silence for a while, then suddenly – Mom looked at me, her glasses slightly askew. "Are you dating?"

"No. I'm too busy for a social life."

"Well, you should be dating someone. I don't understand why a wonderful man hasn't snatched you up."

It was the nicest compliment she had paid me in years. My throat filled with the tears of daily missing Mom, of not being able to call her and discuss my latest book, of no longer sharing a shopping trip or the latest crochet pattern or the encouragement of a Psalm.

"Thanks, Mom. That's nice."

"Well, I'm just askin'."

For a few hours on a hot July afternoon, Mom and I connected on a level long past. She was again the bossy mother, demanding answers and commanding me in directions she wanted me to take.

Once again, I was the daughter and our roles were clear, not reversed or confused in the dynamics of what Alzheimer's does to families.

And for a few hours, we sat together in peace, two women – still joined by an emotional umbilical cord.

Such a sweet moment may never happen again.

EMOTIONAL CAREGIVING

It happens every time.

As soon as I turn away from Mom's door in assisted living and walk down the hallway – away from her, the emotions hit me. After all these years, surely I should accept these raw woundings. Shouldn't this constant grieving have already become my comfort zone?

For ten years my family struggled with Dad's dementia and all the accompanying emotions. Now that Mom has been diagnosed with Alzheimer's, I should expect a similar roller coaster of feelings.

But still – the emotions grip my soul and I cry all the way to the car – then sit in the driver's seat until my vision no longer blurs.

When we become caregivers, certain emotions come to live with us. One of these emotions is sadness. The Long Goodbye, aka Alzheimer's, triggers a sadness unlike any other grief I have suffered.

It is not the unexpected grief of a sudden loss – a miscarriage, unemployment or illness – but rather a day-by-day grief caused by the regressive nature of the disease.

Even though Mom remembers me today, she will someday forget how to introduce me to her friends in assisted living. Sad, but true.

Another sadness lies ahead. If Mom does not graduate to heaven within the next few years, we will have to relocate her to the nursing home section of the facility.

"Never put me in a nursing home." I hear the echo of her plea.

Sadness reinforces the truth that at the end of this particular journey, my siblings and I will be orphans. Grief will multiply as we decorate the tombstones of both parents.

Another emotion, rejection, surfaces every time Mom forgets a memory that is important to me. "Remember when?" is no longer a game we play. And when Mom does hesitate with my name, rejection swallows logic.

I know she does not mean to reject me. Somewhere, cached in her soul is my baby face, her firstborn. But I miss our shopping trips and the way we used to talk about the books we were reading.

I no longer hear her laughter, because she no longer comprehends jokes. When she shows me the greeting cards I sent, clearly imprinted with my signature, then tells me they are from someone else – I feel rejected.

Although sadness and rejection are the emotions that bring fresh pain, guilt is the emotion that tortures me.

No, Mom, we never wanted to put you into assisted living, but you couldn't live alone anymore. All of us work long hours. None of us can take care of you. I'm sorry and I hate it. I feel guilty.

When I hug her goodbye and tell her I have to go back to Kansas, she does not understand why I am leaving. Reality screams that my work is a state away, and my life cannot make room for my mother.
I am the long-distance caregiver in the family, demoted by miles and the work I cannot do anywhere else.
Guilty again.

Even while writing this post, I feel guilty that my emotions are front and center while Mom deals bravely – day after long day – with her own fears, rejection and sadness.

It helps to journal about these caregiving emotions or vent with a friend. These feelings are now my reality, and I know they affect me deeply because they are foreshadowed by love.

If I did not love my mother so much, I would not care. Grief, rejection and guilt would not scar me.

But because I love her, I am sad she cannot be who she used to be.

THE BLESSING OF CLARITY

We sit together in church, my mother holding her Bible – because that is what we do in church. She is no longer able to search for her favorite passages or even comprehend the Table of Contents that would help her locate, "The Lord is my Shepherd."

Yet she is present, because this is a Sunday and this is what we do every Sunday – even within the uncertain shadows.

The horrid disease of Alzheimer's cannot take away our Sunday traditions – at least…not yet. We will worship, then return home to prepare the family dinner. We will eat together – my siblings and I, the grandchildren and my mother – the matriarch who raised us to appreciate this day. We will talk about the past week and the coming week. Then we will take holy naps and praise the God who gives us work on the other six days.

Yet while we sit in golden oak pews, I thank God on this particular day, my mother still comprehends some of what is said and occasionally joins in the songs, especially the old hymns with familiar melodies and safe theology.

I watch her from the corner of my eye. This is the woman who made sure I learned my Sunday school verses. She is the one who drove me to the Good News Club where I fell in love with Jesus and decided to become a Christian. She was the first person I told about my salvation moment, and she rejoiced with me.

I wonder how long she prayed for that moment to become a reality. Did she begin praying on the day she confirmed her pregnancy? Or did she wait until I slithered from her womb and screamed my entrance into the world?

How do I reciprocate those prayers now?

I pray for God's mercy and ask for just a bit of clarity, for the dark shadows of Alzheimers to leave her alone so she can worship on this day, one more Sunday.

The pastor asks for introductions of visitors. He knows my mother struggles with memory yet he pushes her, forces her to remember. "And who is sitting next to you?" he asks.

Every muscle in my body tenses. Will she be able to speak my name – to introduce me? Will she need to think about it for heart-gripping moments while everyone waits? Will she feel obligated to make up a name for me, the person who looks like a younger version of herself?

Ah, yes! She rapidly and clearly answers, "Why, this is my daughter…Rebecca."

Everyone smiles. My heart leaps with joy. On this particular Sunday, on this heat-encrusted August day in Oklahoma…my mother still knows who I am.

FINDING LEGACIES WITHIN ALZHEIMER'S

Because October is my birthday month, my autumn thoughts often center around the woman who raised me. Although Dad reflected the prominent faith figure in my growing-up years, it was Mom who pushed me out of the birth canal, then encouraged me to become who I am.

She was a fighter and an extrovert, unlike the rest of us introverts who disappeared within our private worlds to write, listen to music or find our energy in the solitude of Oklahoma's beauteous landscape.

Odd that I speak of Mom in the past tense, even though her brave heart still beats as she stares at the wall opposite her chair.

That's what Alzheimer's does to a family. We say goodbye one stage at a time, one regression after another so that when death finally releases our loved one – much of the grieving has already completed its course.

Mom grew up poor, walked to high school (yes, miles away, even in the snow and rain) and wore the same two dresses until her Sunday dress became too worn for church. It was then relegated for school wear as her mother sewed a better one for the Sabbath or one of the cousins passed down a Sunday outfit that wasn't yet worn out.

As part of her legacy, Mom was determined none of her children would ever be ashamed of their clothes or feel embarrassed because they didn't fit in. So she learned how to sew, spread out the material on the farmhouse floor, cut, pinned and put together whatever clothes we needed to look like we had some cash in the bank.

Then she made certain each of us understood the importance of a quality education so we would never feel the sting of poverty. We grew up with a solid work ethic, attended college, saved our pennies and never bought anything we didn't really need.

It was a simpler time – a beautiful segment of history, without traffic snarls, school shootings or adultery in every family tree.

I miss it every day.

Mom was willing to live in an old farmhouse and fix it up gradually, spreading wallpaper in rooms that were never plumb and restoring old pieces of furniture to match the country decor. Much of our house mirrored the early-attic variety, but none of us minded. It was a safe place to grow up although cold in the winter and hot in the summer. But who minded when the kitchen smelled like fresh-baked bread, the fields sprouted a golden harvest that supported us all year and the animals taught us about life and death?

As a registered nurse, Mom followed the habits of "old school" nursing. Always dressed in white, her uniform and hat starched and gleaming, her white shoes and hose the perfect accessory. In those days, no jewelry was allowed except a simple wedding band.

But Mom, a bit of a secret radical, wore a cross necklace under her slip. "To remind me I'm a Christian," she said. "To keep me focused on what matters when I have to clean someone's bottom or tell a family their child just died."

Strength of character. Rock solid faith. Those qualities hard to imagine in the woman who now rocks back and forth and accuses visitors of stealing her digital clock.

Yet her strength taught me how to work well even when no one is watching, how to pray my guts out, how to deal with life when it hurts by working hard and moving forward, how to fight against traditions based on men's interpretations rather than the powerful voice of God.

Even now, when I journey through faith crises and wonder how to fit in a church that will accept my calling – I know Mom would understand. If I could just communicate with her, that steely gleam would return to her eyes and she would tell me, "Stop whining. Just get busy and do it."

She was probably one of the first in her generation who envisioned the concept of giving children roots and wings. She taught us well, then let us go and cheered whether we succeeded or learned hard life lessons through failure.

Never demonstrative with her love, if anyone attacked her kids – they faced the wrath of a woman who knew how to struggle through the worst of life's catastrophes and conquer them through sheer grit.

No one dared beat up her kids, either emotionally or physically. She stood tall in her 5'8" frame and declared, "One more word, and I'll jerk a knot in you."

I am proud of the legacy Mom shared with me, strength of character that dares to question the establishment yet humbly accepts God's will.

Even within the shadows of Alzheimer's, I see Mom's resolve to finish her course well, to find contentment in the every dayness of Bingo, planned meals and assigned seats during movie night. The rules of assisted living.

The strong woman who raised me still exists somewhere deep, even though the outer shell gains fragility, age spots and graying hairs.

The legacy continues. Thanks, Mom.

FORSAKE ME NOT

She devoted the major part of 15 years caring for my dad. As he slipped into the silent world of dementia and then Alzheimer's, Mom sat on his lap and spoon-fed him. She sipped from their joint coffee cup, then shared some of the brew with the love of her life.

Every 36-hour day, she fed him, turned him, bathed him and asked God to heal him. Then her prayer concluded with a final selah, "Oh, God. Please don't let me get Alzheimer's."

After we buried Dad, she lived within a five-year respite before her memory started to slip. We noticed it in segments – the same questions asked over and over, the loss of time and space, the forgetting of familiar faces.

Her diagnosis hounded us. How could it be both parents would be afflicted with tragic mental diseases? Was it because of the farm chemicals we used to ensure a harvest year after year? Was it nutrition – too many carbs and not enough fresh veggies? Or was it just the roll of the die and some part of God's plan for the genetics of our family?

I've wondered if King David's parents disappeared into the shadows. Psalm 27:10 records a sad lament from the sensitive heart of the giant-killer, "*Although my father and my mother have forsaken me, yet the Lord will take me up (adopt me as his child).*"

Forsaken, forgotten, cached back in time to some memory before the present. That is the scrapbook my mother now lives – the same story my father lived.

We children who swelled her belly and slithered from her womb have become the enemy. She doesn't understand we want to help her by taking away the car keys and the wallet and the trusting heart that opens the door to every stranger. She forgets when I call and throws away my notes, then tells the neighbors I no longer care. She has forsaken me, just as my father did – though neither of them wanted to.

As I watch Mom disappear into this horrendous valley, my only comfort is that Jesus understands. He was forsaken, too, by family members who did not understand his destiny. Christ knew what it felt like to be rejected and forgotten – if only for a period of time.

He understands how I feel at the gradual loss of my mother – this wretched forsaking. Yet knowing him brings me a measure of hope.

Christ will never forget who I am.

FINDING A LOVE LANGUAGE

In his best-selling book, Gary Chapman explains the love languages as: affection or touch, giving special gifts, spending quality time, acts of service and affirming words.

When we know the love languages of those around us, we can better relate to them.

Growing up in a time and culture where no one ever said, "I love you," we never considered the love languages of family members. We had no idea how important they were.

But now that Mom walks through the shadows of Alzheimer's, I seek ways to communicate with her. Finding her love language is one of my attempts to somehow make a connection.

Receiving gifts is definitely not Mom's love language. When someone gives her something, she loses it and then accuses nurses, grandchildren or visitors of stealing it. Even when she wins a Snickers bar at Bingo, she immediately gives it away. Her life no longer exists in possessions, so gifts are not Mom's love language.

Touch has never been an important facet of our family life. Although Mom will receive my hugs now, she never initiates them. And even within our hugs, when I feel her thin flesh, the vertebrae that march down her spine, warmth is lacking. Touch does not work as a love language for my mother.

Affirming words might be slightly closer for Mom's love language, but not for long. If I say anything nice to her, "Your hair looks really nice today, Mom" or "That color of lavender looks so good against your white hair," she will say thank you and change the subject – or give me one of those looks that means, "You're kidding, right?"

Acts of service. My family has always stressed a strong work ethic. We toiled long and hard, as much for others as for ourselves. Fixing a meal for a shut-in, helping a sick neighbor finish his harvest or baking mounds of banana bread for Christmas gifts – work became an act of love.

But performing an act of service at this juncture in Mom's life would be empty and wasted energy. She would turn it around and want to do something in return for me – if she could, if she dared.

Besides, what act of service can I do for her now? Her laundry is taken care of at the facility. Someone else cooks her meals and serves them to her on beautiful plates. She walks to the salon to have her hair fixed. Her needs are all met.

The only love language that remains is quality time. This is the one way I can show her my love, spending time with her whenever possible. Quality time means sitting in her apartment and answering the same questions over and over without becoming grumpy about it.

It means looking through the cards she has received and talking about the senders of those cards – old friends and new friends, relatives and church members.

It means walking around the pond with her and stopping frequently so she can catch her breath. It means carving some time into a weekend to visit Mom even if neither of us has anything to say.

Loving Mom now means spending time with her. And I'm glad to do it – while I can – before our time together finally ends.

SEEKING THE LIGHT

During Christmas break, I sit in Mom's house, a mile away from the assisted living where she lives. Her house now a shell of what it once was. Her absence a reminder that what we experienced in her house has faded into a new existence – her world within Alzheimer's.

Shadows dance across the walls. Sunset in Oklahoma still wins as my favorite part of the day.

I once climbed my special tree on the family farm, perched alone with my journal in a nest of branches that safely held me. As I watched and worshipped, the turquoise sky framed the wheat field into a portrait of orange, blue and red.

Now within Mom's empty house, I worship the creator of a new sunset as it changes a taupe wall to a natural painting of shadow on light.

The shadows grow deeper for Mom even as they lengthen for my siblings and I. We observe Mom's confusion and recognize more signs of the coming stages.

Our world changes once again as memory fades and communication alters.

Like the sunset that evolves every few minutes, so our family's life is now flexible. We must readily accept each new frame.

Another 24 hours is spent, and I wonder about my own life, my personal calendar of events.

How should I live so that each sunset brings with it a contentment that I lived this day well, that I finished my course with joy and purpose?

How can I live as my own shadows lengthen and deepen, so that the light I have shared will be what is remembered – my legacy to the world and to my son?

None of us is certain of our timelines. We can only attempt to do our best, to live and love and work with pride, to complete the tasks before us and honor the One who gives us the energy to work, to live and love.

We can only commit to a stronger and higher calling so that when sunset comes, we will rejoice in the light that dances at the end of day.

GRIEVING IN SMALL STEPS

One day I met a woman whose son had died in a tragic car accident. One minute he was alive with plans for a wonderful future. The next minute, he lay in a coffin. A terrible event with intense grief.

For families with loved ones who suffer from Alzheimer's, the grief comes in small steps. We know the end of the story and while we don't have any idea what day our loved one will graduate to heaven – we do know the end will come.

But the grief may not be as intense as it was for the sorrowing mother I met.

Alzheimer's grief comes and goes with each regression into the disease. "The Long Goodbye" becomes "The Continual Grief."

Our most intense grief happened at the initial diagnosis. Because our family lived through Dad's dementia, we had an idea of what we faced with Mom. Once that MRI came back with its definitive image, we acknowledged the truth about Mom's future and the grieving began.

My first grief step was anger. How completely unfair that my mother should be sentenced to this horrible disease. Where was the just God she loved so much? Questions revealed no answers. Easy solutions morphed into daily routines of just trying to endure it.

Then came the sadness, one tiny piece at a time: when Mom could no longer find her pots and pans in the kitchen, when she forgot to eat, when we had to make the decision to put her into assisted living.

Each decision evoked its own realm of sadness. The grief merged into a quilted pattern of daily struggle while the only hope was that it might not last as long as Dad's dementia. Wrong assumption.

I know what some of the next steps of grief will look like: when Mom forgets who I am, when she crosses that line of communication where she can no longer speak, when we have to move her into the nursing home area of the building, when we pick out her final outfit and sign the papers at the mortuary.

As horrible as it sounds, for caregivers that final grief is actually a release. When our loved one finally graduates to heaven and we know their minds are suddenly clear, we're happy for them.

Our day-to-day sadness turns to joy because we know the sounds of the long good-bye have finally merged into glorious hallelujahs.

Grief is difficult, no matter how it happens – whether intense moments or bit and pieces. None of us grieves in the same way and no one can tell us how to do it well. We have to find our way through that tunnel alone.

But one thing we do know – all of us at one time or another *will* grieve. We will feel the emotions of loss during our time on earth.

The trick is to somehow find hope in the midst of that unraveling and be grateful for the life our loved ones have lived.

Grief means we have experienced love and whether it comes all at once or in small steps – acknowledging the love restores hope.

FINDING HOPE IN THE DARK

It was a subtle change, yet I felt its impact as if a door slammed shut in my heart.

During the Thanksgiving weekend, I visited Mom. Each of the three days when I knocked and entered her room, Mom sat in her chair – in the dark.

Alone – with a book on her lap, pretending to read.

Just a few months ago, I often found her at a table with other residents, playing cards – laughing together, competing and exercising their brain cells.

Not this time. The Long Goodbye had moved into another stage of memory loss.

Others still played in the dining hall. They shuffled cards and tossed them at each other, then laughed at their silliness, enjoying the camaraderie of the game.

But they played without my mother, and I wondered why.

After several moments trying to communicate with her, I realized the reason she sat alone, sans an activity she once enjoyed.

She doesn't play cards anymore because she can't. The comprehension required for something as simple as Rook or Uno no longer exists. Numbers, sequences and patterns now fail to make a connection. Even the fun of being with other residents cannot replace the inactivity of brain cells.

So my mother sits in the dark, woven within herself.

I joined her there, rarely speaking, but sharing the shadows as two women. One of us not comprehending the subtraction of comrades. The other grieving at another piece of lost aliveness.

An hour later, I drove away, then pulled over, beating the steering wheel and crying out to the God who allowed this dark loneliness to invade my mother's life.

So unfair. Such an emptiness in what was once a full life.

But then I remembered the book Mom held on her lap during our time together, the words she read over and over, even without comprehending.

Her Bible.

Even though Alzheimer's deletes entertaining card games and clouds the comprehension needed for winning – Mom still knows where to find hope.

She is never truly alone because Emanuel lives within her, loving her through this journey and offering his light in her darkness.

WHEN HUMOR EASES THE JOURNEY

When our children are little, we keep a journal of their cute sayings, their trials with language and their funny mistakes. We laugh and share these moments with grandparents and any friends who will listen.

When our parents become children because of plaque-laden Alzheimer's, we still laugh at their funny stories. These moments aren't as cute at age 80+, but laughter provides the necessary impetus to make it through another caregiving day.

So when I share the funny things Mom has done, I'm not mocking her or making fun of her. I hope to encourage other caregivers, to share a common bond and to keep humor as one of our coping mechanisms.

Last week, Mom lost her bobby pins. Although she is scheduled for the salon each week, she still fixes her hair every night with tiny curls held in place with bobby pins. And she carries a small sack of bobby pins in her pocket. I don't know why. For some reason, bobby pins are her connection with a former life.

Keeping as many routines as possible is an important part of coping with Alzheimer's. So we don't mind when Mom manages to curl a section of her still-thick white hair and pin it securely. Even if we are on our way to church and her hair looks great. Even if we are sitting in the dark and no one cares about hair styles.

But this week, the vital bobby pins were missing and Mom was convinced they were stolen. "Someone comes into my room at night. And while I'm sleeping, they steal my bobby pins right off my head."

The visual of this possibility nearly knocks me to the floor with laughter. The mystery of the Bobby Pin Burglar and his goal of stealing the curls from my mother's head.

The bobby pin story kept us laughing for a while, until Mom lost her bridge and the teeth attached to it. In spite of an application of extra cement by the dentist, Mom managed to loosen her bridge, yank it out of her mouth and then lose it.

Again she was convinced, "Someone stole my teeth."

My sister asked, "Why would someone steal your teeth? What would they do with them?"

Always ready with an answer, Mom said, "They'll take them to the dentist and trade my teeth for new dentures."

A creative vision flashed through my mind of a homeless woman. She carried a plastic sack filled with stolen teeth, including my mother's bridge. The woman combed through her hair, trying to make herself feel more decent and somehow accepted by the professionals in the dentist's office.

She walked through the door and asked, "How much will you give me for these? I need dentures and I'm trying to save money."

Stares. Someone called 9-1-1 and the homeless shelter. No one offered to make the exchange. The woman returned to the streets, still carrying her sack of stolen teeth.

My mother's active imagination and propensity for losing things gave a new significance to the finding of humor in the journey.

We laugh because we dare not cry. Too many tears will drown us in despair.

I CAN'T STAND IT

It happened again this week. I heard someone say, "God won't give us more than we can bear."

This is theologically and biblically incorrect yet many people believe it. No doubt they are misinterpreting First Corinthians 10:13 where Paul writes, *"No temptation has overtaken you but such as is common to man; and God is faithful, who will not allow you to be tempted beyond what you are able, but with the temptation will provide the way of escape also, that you may be able to endure it."*

God does not allow us to be tempted above what we can bear. He provides an escape so we can have victory over the many things that tempt us and prevent them from becoming strongholds.

But God does not promise we will not experience trial after trial and horror so difficult we cannot bear it. In fact, God didn't even do that for his son, Jesus, who cried out "Why?" from the cross.

Holocaust victims, sex trafficking victims, burn victims – who of us can bear that kind of pain? Yet God allowed it.

For some reason he has allowed the disease of Alzheimer's to invade our world. Family dynamics change. Parents forget their children and the security of a homestead peopled with precious grandparents disappears.

I can't stand it.

What God does promise is that his grace is sufficient, no matter what we're going through. This is not the saving grace that rescues us from an eternity in hell. Rather, it is the powerful grace that lends strength when we're going through hell on earth. When we're living through the emotional furnace of Alzheimer's and dementia.

God sometimes allows us to go through situations that we – in our own strength – cannot deal with. We cannot bear it on our own, and we cannot find the grit within us to keep smiling.

We need God's powerful stamina, his strengthening grace. He allows us things we cannot bear to encourage us to move away from our self-sufficiency and depend on him.

If my mother could converse, she might cry out, "I can't stand it. I cannot bear the forgetting of my children's names or the loss of my ability to pray. I will not be able to stand it when I lose all sensibilities and someone will have to diaper me, cleanse me and roll me over. I cannot stand this Alzheimer's journey."

The one blessing of this disease is that the victim eventually reaches a level where she is unaware of what is happening to her. She prays in an inner place of cached memories while her caregivers deal with the daily grind of caring for her.

Caregivers are the ones now crying out, "I can't stand it."

Mom has always known she needed the powerful hand of God to uphold her during the times he allowed more than she could bear: the loss of grandchildren born before they could survive, a plentiful harvest disappearing in the green clouds of sudden hail, when Alzheimer's stole her ability to work, when she could no longer drive.

Yet she bore those situations with courage and continued to live in hope.

It is now our place, as her children and caregivers, to put into action the lessons she taught us, to focus on God's strength.

It is our role to ask for God's help when we absolutely cannot stand the Alzheimer's journey one more moment.

In the acknowledgement of our need, God proves he can always and forever deal with it. He can bear it when we cannot.

FINDING HOPE IN BIRTHDAYS

October, 2014, signified more than just another month flipped past on the calendar. It was my birthday month, the time I set aside once a year to evaluate who I have become and which goals I will set for the next year. Even as I age, Octobers still hold the promise of more life to experience, more books to write, more spiritual growth to strive for.

But the 2014 October carried more meaning for me than just a celebration, a reason to allow myself some dark chocolate mixed with fresh blueberries. It represented all the birthdays Mom made special through all the years. I waited for her call even though I knew it may not come. Would she remember the day?

My heart blipped when I reached into the mailbox and pulled out the envelope – the obvious size for a greeting card – the return address from Enid, Oklahoma.

Mom. She was late, but she remembered.

Inside the card was a check for twenty dollars. But as I read the card with its stamped violets and a naughty kitten peeking out from behind a watering can, I peered at the check. Something surprising and terrible. Almost immediately, I beat my fists on the kitchen counter and began to sob.

Mom had tried to write her signature on the check, but obviously crossed out her name and rewrote it, then printed her initials to indicate the change. This was no mistake, no slipping of the fingers or pen. It was another sign of regression – another step downward into the pit of Alzheimer's.

I remembered how Dad, slipping into dementia, sat at the table and practiced the alphabet. He was beginning to forget his name yet wanted so desperately to remember. So he started at the beginning – relearning his a-b-c's. A grown man trying to concentrate, to make the simple letters he had known for eighty years.

Heartbreaking. The forgetting of words and numbers – a side effect of Alzheimer's.

Now my mom struggled to write her name, scratching it out and trying again to create the signature she had carried for a lifetime. It was a reminder how the time bomb of Alzheimer's ticks away and each change signifies another stage of this dreaded disease.

How could I search for hope, knowing the downward spiral we traveled? Beyond the now stale birthday cake, the collection of cards displayed on the piano's lid and the shiny Mylar balloon drooping as helium slowly escaped.

Another day ended. Another descent into Mom's disease.

I took a deep breath and found hope in the one place where it is constantly nurtured and harvested – the book of Psalms. "*When I am old and gray, O God, you will not forsake me, until I have shown your strength to this generation and your power to everyone that is to come*" (Psalm 71:18).

Even though Mom's brain betrayed her and her fingers with their memorized motions forsook her – God was still evident in her life. His love reflected in her smile when she saw me walk through the door. He was the Comforter when she forgot someone's name and solved the problem with a cheerful, "Hi there, Kid." He was the answer when she stared into space and repeated the same questions over and over.

He is omniscient, the one who knows the timeline of her life – how many days are left and how they will play out.

God still showed his strength through Mom because when I saw the regression, I was forced to acknowledge his powerful presence.

Somehow the God who owns our hearts would hold us close throughout this horrific disease. Somehow he would create a way for us to cope and help us emit a strong yet tender grace for Mom throughout the next stages of the disease.

Even within the sorrow of my birthday, I found hope because I knew God would not forsake us. He would comfort us throughout the final stages of the journey and beyond.

Mom may not be able to sign her full name, but Someone – who has recorded every hair on her head – will never forget her. And he will hold all of us in the palm of his mighty hand as we continue to find our hope in him.

TELEVISION BECOMES A COMPANION

As I entered assisted living and walked down the hallway, I heard the blaring sound and wondered, *Is that Mom's television? Surely not.*

But as I knocked on the door, the noise of the McDonald's commercial hit me like notes galloping through musical cyberspace.

Mom sat in her maroon recliner, watching but not really comprehending the images. "The Idiot Box," she always called it. Yet here she was, mesmerized by its siren call of soap operas, commercials and baseball games of teams she did not recognize.

Television was never a revered object on the farm. In fact, Mom turned off the set after the evening news so my siblings and I could finish our homework. When chores and homework were finished, we chose another book from the stack of library books on the coffee table. Our nightly regimen always included chores, homework and reading.

The only sound in the house came from the old stereo playing one of Dad's classical albums. "Victory at Sea" was a favorite although Dad and I had a special affinity for Beethoven's Ninth. "Joyful joyful we adore thee, God of glory, Lord of love."

I hummed the chorus as I lay on my stomach by the fireplace, a book opened before me, my black and white Oxford shoes waving with the rhythm of the chords.

A television show that could never compete with the musical genius of Beethoven.

The symphony of farm life reverberated into the past as I turned down the volume on Mom's television set. No silence here. Its cacophony interrupted not only our visit but also boomed its sound down the hallway and into the rooms of other residents.

Such a rude instrument. I understood why Mom was so insistent that our evenings on the farm were never filtered with television's influence.

Whether from boredom, loneliness or the need to have something of humanity in her room, Mom now turns to the television for companionship. With her hearing slowly declining, she ups the volume, then collapses into the numbing comfort of her recliner.

Oblivious to the national news. Not caring about the weather reports. The staff at the assisted living will tell Mom if a tornado heads her way, if a hail storm pelts the one window in her studio apartment.

She ignores my presence in the room and once again turns up the volume to Scream level. Although enraptured in the images that play across the television screen, Mom admits, "I hate the TV. I'd rather read a book."

She points to one of the many books she reads over and over again, reaches for a Reader's Digest condensed version and opens it. Occasionally, she looks at me and asks one of the many questions we have already discussed.

I pull my own book out of my bag and disappear into the words while agreeing with Mom about our hatred of the blaring instrument across the room.

The core values of the Alzheimer's patient do not always coincide with their behavior. What the heart and mind believe does not always jibe with action. Mom hates the television, yet craves the noise of its presence.

It is another reminder of the difficulties of communication. When Alzheimer's overshadows a behavior inconsistent with life's memory, we seek patience and another level of understanding.

The noisemaker in the room is now Mom's companion, but it will never replace the life story of this woman who read voraciously and made sure her children learned to love books.

When I returned home, I ignored the screen in the corner and refused to tune into the weather report. Instead, I opened my journal to record more thoughts about Mom.

It seemed a fitting memorial.

GOING THROUGH TRIALS ALONE

Some things must be borne alone.

Although we enlist the prayers of other saints and feel the power of their intercession, we still travel through the trials alone. Somehow we must find our own courage to deal with the struggle of Alzheimer's and learn to cope – each family finding their own pathway to hope.

Yes…God is with us. He promises to never leave us. But when we lie on sterile tables and allow the dermatologist to shave skin off our mortal bodies, we feel alone with the fear of wondering, *Is it melanoma? Will he get all the tissue and scrape away the mess of toxic cells?*

We endure the pressure of a mammogram and pray everything will be all right but in those moments of hanging on to metal while the pain takes away breath – we are alone with the brutality of the machine. Even the radiologist hides behind a safe partition and quietly reads the screen that can change the number of our days.

As parents, we want to rescue our children from trials. But we are as helpless as the screaming infants laid on our bare stomachs, bloody from the sac and screaming from the umbrage of a contracting birth canal.

Our children grow and we wait in emergency rooms, knowing a beloved son is behind that steel door – alone in his own trial. We struggle to believe for the best yet wait alone with the fear.

We live through the hardest moments alone, hoping God in his mercy will grant us a special measure of grace to live it courageously.

How can we prepare for the journey of Alzheimer's – when our loved one struggles alone and each of us in the family deals with our own dynamics in a single-minded knot of determination? How can we make it through this journey and come out on the other side without the ravages of stress, a mass of newly-grayed hair or wrinkles that now mark us as children of the Long Goodbye?

We Prepare Now. When times are still good or at least reasonably bearable, we spend time getting to know God better. We stock up on Bible promises and fill the molecules of air around our beds with multiple prayers. Just as we sweat through the plank or other core-strengthening exercises, we now build up spiritual muscles – for later – when we are alone.

Community Strength. We surround ourselves with a community of others. Whether a group of saints who know how to pray or a special group we trust, we surround the days with people who will be with us when we wake up from surgery, when the steel door shuts behind the gurney, when the mammogram comes back positive, when the diagnosis is Alzheimer's. We build relationships now to encourage us later.

Live in Gratitude. If this is not a day for struggle, we enjoy the sunshine and touch the dew on the roses. We journal thoughts and take pictures we can relish when we're faced with the unbelievable. We make each day a Hallmark expression of gratitude so hope will not quickly fade into despair. When the tough times come, we will then be practiced at looking for something good even within the pain.

A day will arrive when the trial lifts and we will return to peaceful joy. We hang on to hope in the now and prepare for the days when aloneness is our only companion.

RESPECTING THE ALZHEIMER'S PATIENT

A blog post was already written, edited and almost scheduled. Then I had second thoughts.

It was a post about my mother and shared one of the family secrets she told me years ago. I knew it was a great post, and I hoped it would interest my followers as well as give them insights into the life of my mother.

But somehow – I could not post it.

Mom is an extrovert but she has also been a private person, hiding her secrets in a sacred soul place. That's what women in her demographic learned to do. That's how she taught us to live as well.

In today's world of vulnerability and Brene Brown TED talks, stuffing our secrets has proven unhealthy. We share our true selves with those we trust. We learn to own our pain, admit its core and move forward in life.

But in Mom's world, that never happened. Never would she have shared her life via social media nor would she want me to do that for her by proxy. I respect that private piece of her personality and choose to keep aspects of her life – and ultimately my family's life – cached in its secret vault.

As a curious adolescent, I snooped in Mom's hope chest and read the beautiful love letters my parents wrote to each other. While I reveled in finding out how human my parents were, I felt guilt for the intrusion into their love life – their younger selves – before they welcomed me into their inner circle.

Other family secrets were told by caring and not-so-caring relatives through the years. Doesn't every family have that uncle or aunt who won't shut up – the relative who embarrasses everyone yet is still mourned when the coffin slowly descends into summer-baked soil?

As an adolescent writer, my instinct was to explore some of the more private stories, to write a family memoir and encase it in a time capsule for posterity. When I asked Mom to explain missing pieces of our history, she pursed her lips and changed the subject.

Off limits – even though I was family.

Even now, as my siblings and I age, as cousins spread across the nation and we no longer gather for reunions, those stories remain as tidbits of experience. We were told some of the plot lines, but without the character sketches I so love as a now grownup writer.

Yet knowing how to write still does not give me license to share with the world all about my mother's life.

I will simply write that she lived life well. She raised three children and loved her husband with all her heart. She served as a nurse, baked bread every weekend, planned harvest meals and managed to keep the food warm even when the farmer and his field hands were late – trying to eek that last kernel from the wheat head before storms pelted our annual income from its source.

Mom inspected our ears after baths, paid for piano lessons and drove us to the city pool to learn how to swim. She spread Simplicity patterns across the floor and cut out pieces of cloth, then sewed them together so we had something new for the first day of school. In the winter months, out came her crochet needle and colorful skeins of yarn. By the end of February, another afghan decorated one of our beds or draped across Dad's club chair by the fireplace.

One year, she came home pale with her eyes rimmed from fresh tears. "What's wrong," I asked, afraid that a relative had crossed into the heavenly beyond.

"Oh, work," she said. "A woman came in to have her baby. It should have been simple, but she died. I had to tell her husband."

After that bombshell, Mom blew her nose and retreated silently to the back porch where she proceeded to defrost the freezer. Later in life, I learned the different ways people grieve. Some are emotional while others – like my mom and most of my siblings – are industrial. When we grieve, we get busy and do something. We work to relieve the pain.

So I will not add to my mother's grief by telling any of her deepest secrets. I will keep those plot lines to myself and reserve the memoir of my life for my son, telling what I wish yet preserving what I must.

Because I respect Mom and the life she lived, I will keep her secrets in that sacred place of the soul – a pact between us no one else needs to know.

I love you, Mom.

CEMETERY WANDERINGS

My personal tradition calls for a visit to the cemetery during Easter weekend. Somehow, the credibility of the resurrection needs to meet with the mortality of my ancestors. My faith requires a concrete representation of the living Christ.

Ours is a Mennonite cemetery, on the same acre of land as the old hand-built church, crafted by men who wore beards and black hats. This sacred space contains the remains of generations of Mennonites who traveled to this land of freedom so they could worship freely. These carpenters and farmers now lie below the soil, under rich dirt that grows hard red winter wheat just an acre away.

This was the place that represented closure for me, and for some reason – I needed to refire the embers of remembrance.

I don't believe in talking to the dead through a group séance or messing around with a Ouija board, but I often ask God to talk to Dad and others for me. I imagine the saints sitting in chairs like the scene from "Our Town" – that great cloud of witnesses mentioned in the book of Hebrews.

I stopped first at Dad's headstone and laid wildflowers near his name. The engraving already complete for when Mom joins him, sans her final expiration date – a carving of wheat next to Dad's name, flowers next to Mom's. The lifelong love story and commitment of two people who though very different in temperament and personality managed to keep their love fresh for 50 plus years.

"I miss him, God. Tell Dad I'm thinking of him today. I wish he could attend my book signings and read my books. Is there a library in heaven?"

It is his shell I miss. The strum of his fingers on guitar strings, his baritone voice singing "Blessed Assurance," his bow-legged stroll through the pasture on frosty mornings.

"Ah, God...tell Dad I need him to help me past this lonely place in my soul. I long to hear him pray for me once again and find a verse for me in the leather Bible he crafted. I miss having my daddy in my life."

Next I roamed near the gravestone of the woman who introduced me to Jesus. "God, oh God – tell Matilda how much I appreciate her. She told me about your love and helped me understand how to become a Christian. What a wonderful woman she was!

"And God, here is where Lydia's shell lies. She taught Sunday School when I was a little girl, and I remember her being so kind. Tell her thank you, please. She was a sweet reminder of your love.

"Here are the shells of Dan and Alma – neighbors who flew to heaven just eight weeks apart. They loved each other so much, they couldn't stand to be separated. How sweet is that!"

My in-laws, Jake and Leora. "Tell them, God, how much I loved them. I miss them."

The grandparents and great grands I never met. "Do they know about me, God? Are they proud of me? Are you?"

So many babies' graves. In the 1800's, many infants lived only one or two days. Was it SIDS or a childhood illness, something simple like the croup we now easily cure with antibiotics?

I imagined God watching over his heavenly nursery and loving each baby. Two of them are mine. Ryan and Rachel who slithered from my womb too early.

Then once more, I knelt before Dad's grave and brushed winter's dust from the stone surround. A few tears, a soul hurt. "The family will be together soon, Dad – at the farm. I loved being a country girl. Mom is in assisted living. She has Alzheimer's, but I know she misses you. We all do.

"Do you know I'm a published author? Has God told you about my books? Some of your life and your journey is in my books. Those years of dementia, as you struggled to communicate with us and then just stopped talking – I used those experiences in my plots. I wanted caregivers to be encouraged, to know they are doing holy work, caring for their loved ones.

"Ah, Dad – I miss you so much."

Too many tears shed over this grave. I walk again through the cemetery of my ancestors. So much history in this place. So many untold stories which only the Alpha and Omega knows.

Names of Sunday School teachers and pastors, of twins who lived only one day – a tiny sheep engraved next to their names. Vets from the World Wars and Korea lying beside veterans of the faith.

A solitary grave near the wheat field. Another baby – this one died in 1930. But fresh flowers point heavenward next to the aging stone. Who has been here to remember this child?

A wind rippled through the cedars that bordered the cemetery. All alone in the place of legacy and influential lives, I sang that old Easter hymn, "Lo in the grave he lay, Jesus my Savior. Waiting the coming day, Jesus my Lord...he arose, he arose. Hallelujah Christ arose."

As I left the cemetery, I added my own hallelujahs, anticipating the day when those graves would open, the bodies of saints joining with their souls in heaven and I – thank you, Jesus – would be close behind them.

The creative writer in me longed to stay on this sacred ground and make up stories about each grave, but I was due at the assisted living facility, then on to another booksigning. It was time to visit my mother – to spend hours with the living while possible.

Within this visit to this particular cemetery, I heard a sermon. Each soul who lay in this consecrated plot of land now resided somewhere eternal. The cross displayed on so many of the gravestones a solid reminder of who they believed in and the hope of eternity for all of us.

Although I felt a palpable grief in the rows of cemetery wanderings, I knew this was not the end. On this Easter weekend and every one to come, resurrection claimed the final victory.

DISCOVERING THE SAINTS

When I visited my mother-in-law at her assisted living facility, we talked about the passing of seasons. Besides the obvious winter month of November, Christmas and the season of blizzards – we discussed the particular seasons of life.

Her season now included living in the beautiful and secure setting where she was surrounded by those who helped her remember when lunch was served and when it was time to visit the hair salon.

Her nails had grown long and were carefully manicured because her daughters made sure she received that nurturing treat. During a previous season, I remembered her as the hard-working housewife, puttering around her kitchen with brittle fingernails thrust into dishwater several times a day.

But life was different now. She had no dishes to wash and no floors to scrub, so she grew her nails long and chose any color she wished for the nail tech to paint. Usually a bright red – her favorite.

I was glad for her this tiny yet significant joy.

As I accompanied her to lunch, I looked around and saw faces of my past. The father of one of my high school friends held himself erect even as he slowly made his way through the buffet line. I remembered the quiet dignity of this aging saint, the way he encouraged us to sing, to pray and trust. His hair, once a flaming red, now reflected over 80 years of pigment change while wrinkles lined the face that once smiled at us from a left side pew, half-way

163

down.

Another gentleman recognized me before I recalled his name. He once worked the land as my father did. I remembered one harvest when my family had to leave the fields to attend the funeral of my uncle.

While we were gone, this farmer gathered his family together, left his own fields untended and cut our wheat. A necessary kindness farmers often presented to their neighbors – a way to pay it forward. They knew we would reciprocate if they ever needed the same.

This man stood before me and explained his sad Thanksgiving season. A second son has preceded him to heaven – the backwards motion of life that tragically surprises, reminding us there are no guarantees no matter what our age.

Each day so precious it can never be retrieved.

I saw the grief behind his eyes, yet he managed a smile – a reminder that our shared faith reached much farther than the cemetery filled with mounded graves.

Another saint ate near us. I recognized the gracious woman who once served in various hospitality ministries. She was now confined to a wheelchair and the daughter who tended her wore the same smile, bearing resemblance not only to physical traits but also to the holy inhabitant within.

My mother-in-law finished her lunch, and I managed to snag a piece of pecan pie for her, remembering her own pecan pies during past seasons. I could never replicate her pies, even when I explicitly followed the recipe. I always relied on Mrs. Smith and the frozen varieties to compensate for my lack of culinary finesse.

The seasons of the past flowed around me in the aging faces of faith – these elders who passed on to a young girl the importance of church attendance and scripture memory, the joy of interceding for each other as we loped through worship together.

I felt waves of gratitude for the example of these saints, these living images of the Hebrews 11 heroes and sheroes who whispered advice through the ages. These were the folks who now waited out their timelines in assisted living while I continued in the ministry of my current season.

One season blends into another but each season is affected by the weather of the previous, just as the faith behaviors of these aged saints once affected me.

I could only hope my life would prove to be a favorable influence on the generations younger than I – those who may someday visit me in the winter season of my life.

A LETTER TO MOM

Dear Mom,

This Sunday is Mother's Day, and I sent you a card. Hopefully, you will understand the words and remember who I am from my signature on the bottom. I wish I could be there with you, but since I can't – please know I love you and celebrate Mother's Day with you.

Although I know you may not understand this letter, I needed to write it anyway as a tribute to you and as grief therapy for me.

Because I am grieving, Mom, at the slow disintegration of the woman you used to be. Your Alzheimer's journey has taught me to value each day, love fully those who are in my life and never forget to make that love known.

But you are disappearing piece by fragile piece, and every time I see you – I am more aware of it.

It wasn't until I became a mother that I understood how much of ourselves we pour into our children. And I'm not just talking about the meals, the activities and making chicken soup when we're sick.

I'm talking about the soul-giving mothers extend to their children – as you extended to me.

Everyone knows about the labor and contractions you endured during my birth, but you also labored with soul contractions throughout my growing up years.

When you were bone tired from working your shift at the hospital, you came home to make supper, finished a load of laundry and still made it to my softball game on time. Not once did you complain. In fact, when I looked into the crowd, you were the one cheering loudest for me.

You defended me when other kids or even adults said unkind things. You taught me how to make the perfect zwieback with just the right dimple on top so melted butter pooled inside that crevasse. And you showed me how to sew a perfect hem so no one except the two of us could see the stitches.

I thank you, Mom, for the late nights when I know you were on your knees for me. You poured out your soul to Almighty God and asked him to keep me safe, but at the same time you were willing to let me go and let God do his work in my life.

You seemed proud when I left home to serve as a missionary, and you only cried when I returned – relieved I was safe and grateful for the experience. I know you prayed for me every day and asked God to send some of his big guy warrior angels to protect your daughter so far from home.

Years later, you came to the hospital when I lost my baby – your first grandchild. Even now, I remember coming out of that anesthesia-induced haze. It was your hand that gripped mine – your tears mingling salty with mine.

These days, I grip your hand and try not to cry when you repeat the same questions over and over.

Many experts have written about the unique bond between mothers and daughters. We depend so deeply on each other, filling a particular emotional need no one else can touch. I think you and I are especially close because we share some of the same personality traits, not to mention a love for Jamoca Chocolate anything.

You taught me how to bake bread, using our ancestors' Mennonite recipe, but you also showed me how to test when the bread was ready. Bread dough wears a specific sheen and texture when the kneading ends and the rising begins. I can still bake bread by touch.

You also taught me how to crochet and embroider, making those tiny stitches that look great on both sides of the fabric. Now I make hand-woven gifts and pray a blessing over each project, asking God to touch the heart of the recipient. I think of you whenever I give one of these colorful projects away.

You taught me to love books. You drove me to the library every week so I could check out books and devour them when I finished my chores. Then you provided the perfect example as you sat under the floor lamp and read your own stack of library books.

You still love reading, though you no longer comprehend the words as you read the same book over and over. Another of the sad effects of this demon Alzheimer's.

I am now a published author, Mom. All those years of reading resulted in the birthing of words in my soul. I am hoping my words will encourage caregivers and families going through this travesty.

You wanted to be a writer, and I'm sorry that didn't happen for you. Instead, you nourished the dream of your daughter.

You always insisted I use proper grammar. I still know the difference between further and farther, lay and lie. By assigning me chores on the farm, you taught self-discipline and a strong work ethic. The weeds I pulled in the pecan orchard, the hours I spent milking the cow and helping during wheat harvest – those qualities also play into my writing life.

In fact, today I am using self-discipline to write this book when I would rather be digging in my garden, planting yellow blooms with red centers or reading a book someone else wrote. You taught me the value and joy of planting seeds that result in happiness for many.

I remember your fingers pulling my long hair tight and weaving it into braids. Your skills as a nurse helped keep me healthy, even when I hated taking medicine.

You worked long hours so I could attend the high school of my choice and the college that offered the best education in my field. I graduated without the burden of student loans to haunt me. Thank you for your perseverance, Mom.

You taught me how to save money by ignoring the impulses of my peers. I learned I didn't have to look like everybody else or own the same things as my friends. You showed me how my value lies in who I am rather than in what I own.

Ahead of your time, you taught me women should think ahead and pursue a career, manage their own money and be prepared for whatever life hands us. You said it was okay to vote differently from my friends and even worship in a style different from the norm. You taught me to think independently, to shush the fear and step into the world with self-confidence and courage.

Oh, you weren't perfect, Mom. None of us are. But even then, you taught me perfection is not the goal and failure is not the end.

Rather, the goal is in the attempt and in the perseverance to try again. Then if we fail, we give ourselves grace, grieve a bit and go forward once again. It is in the attempts and the perseverance our character grows, no matter what life throws at us.

So, Mom, on this weekend of remembrance when people buy flowers and send cards – I want you to know you did a good job. You brought me into the world and gave me the freedom to discover my purpose within that world. You encouraged me to use my gifts and showed me it was okay to be a radical, independent woman. You labored and prayed, then feasted on my accomplishments.

And even though life has handed you this lousy disease, you're still trying every day to put one foot before the other and learn contentment in your small apartment at assisted living.

Above all, Mom, I thank you for being so brave and I love you for showing me how.

THE LEARNING OF PATIENCE

As a Christian, I try to focus on the positives in life – those creative surprises God can produce within any situation.

He promises to create something good out of our struggles if we look for the good – if we trust he knows a better way.

Truthfully, this core value has not been easy as I have watched my mother disappear into the shadows of Alzheimer's Disease. This trial seems to bear with it only the negatives, the sorrow and the unending disappearance of memory and identity.

But on days when I feel stronger, I consider what Alzheimer's has taught me. What has been one of the emotional or spiritual benefits? What have I learned by observing this disease even as it gradually takes my mother away?

Patience.

Answering Mom's repeated questions over and over taxes my patience, but then I think about the question from my mother's point of view. For her, it isn't the same question. It's a new query every few minutes.

Each question and answer segment represents a different moment in time. And since time is reconfigured during Alzheimer's, the asking of the same question sort of makes sense – at least from her perspective.

If I stop, breathe and wait for inspiration from God, I sometimes create a new way to answer Mom's questions. Or I change the subject and lead her into a different conversation where we start all over.

It helps me to search for patience when I remember the day will come when Mom's questioning will stop. She will no longer be able to formulate sentences. She will stop speaking entirely, and I will miss the sound of her voice.

While we're both still existing in the present tense, I find the motivation for patience.

When Mom forgets how to put in her hearing aid, I observe the patience of my sister repeating instructions once again. "Put it in your right ear. Push it all the way in. You can do it."

When Mom can't find the slippers we just bought her, patience helps us look for them.

When she no longer knows what day it is, even though we've circled it on the calendar – patience whispers, "Tuesday, Mom. It's still Tuesday."

This disease has changed Mom, so patience also waits while we figure out how to journey through another stage. And in this waiting, we caregivers are also changed.

Patience reminds me of the mother she once was, the many ways she helped me remember to do my homework and take out the trash, reminded me of piano lessons – how she made sure I arrived at church and school on time.

Patience remembers how Mom taught me to tie my shoes, brush my teeth and practice daily on the piano. In return, my heart needs to be patient with her – especially now.

Patience waits for the sunset of another day and hopes this will be that special date on the heavenly calendar when Mom joins Dad and Jesus in heaven.

I strive for patience because that is what God asks me to do. Patience being a fruit of the spirit resides in me yet constantly needs to be enriched.

Surely when Mom hears the frustration in my voice – it hurts her feelings. It hurts God, too.

So I keep trying to learn and exhibit different forms of patience.

Some day the need for patience will end. Mom will no longer respond at all. Yet somewhere, I hope, in the pockets of her memory – she will remember me and smile. She will observe how I'm trying, how I yearn to be patient with her.

May I learn well these lessons of patience, because some day I, too, may need them returned to me.

EACH DAY COUNTS

Although most of us aspire to the philosophy of carpe diem, do we really live every 24 hours to its fullest?

How quickly the focus of our days can change. An email announces the downsizing of a company. A phone call reverberates with the doctor's prognosis. A memory blip signals the beginning of a downward slope.

A few years ago, Mom seemed fine. She paid her bills, drove her car all over town and maintained the care of her house. She remembered birthdays, called me weekly and we carried on long conversations. She competed with fervor when we played board games and often – she won.

Gradually, we noticed the differences in Mom – the forgetfulness, the questions asked over and over, the fear about losing her way when she drove home. Still, she seemed to cope adequately with life. She was able to stay in her own home.

Everything changed so quickly. After her pacemaker surgery, Mom's carpe diem flipped. Was it the result of her surgery, of hours under anesthesia, the trauma of a body invaded?

Worse. The doctor tested her cognitive recognition and said, "She can no longer live alone."

I wanted to go back and relive each day before, to focus on carpe diem before Mom's diagnosis. But we cannot go back to visit regret. We have only these moments of now and what will someday follow.

Because symptoms and the prognosis of life can change quickly, it's important to say "I love you" often, to treasure each visit together, to journal the memories, take pictures and think fondly of times when everyone exists within cognitive health.

Even now, Mom lingers within assisted living where the balance of the daily process hangs on fragility. She could fall or forget how to dress herself. In those moments, her new address would revert to nursing home care where someone would feed her and her bed would become her companion.

This vicious disease has ironically taught me to treasure each day I have with my son, to live the philosophy of carpe diem and dedicate myself to serve God with the time I am given.

Because I know even one piece of amyloidal plaque can totally change a life. One email, one phone call, one bend in the road we did not expect.

It is within these moments of time God is most mysterious, because he is beyond the ticking of clocks or the flipping over of digital numbers. He is Beginning and End and everything in between, Alpha and Omega, forever and ever. He is the great I am, the maker of time and seasons, the designer of brains and beating hearts.

As the great I am, he simply is – the designer who exists within a passive verb yet actively plans each nanosecond of our lives. The One whose carpe diem chimes eternal, beyond understanding or human measurement.

My faith reaches out to the concept of eternity where clocks and planners will not remind us of important meetings, where flowers will bloom forever and death will never interrupt.

But until we reach that place of abstract where time as we know it fades, our role is to treasure each second together. Each day so precious, because it is all we have.

MAKING POSITIVE MEMORIES

When our memories begin to deteriorate, we will want our children and other family members to remember good things about our time together.

Life can be so busy with work, school and more work – with paying bills, facing conflict and defeating fear. But in the midst of all the hubbub, we can determine to make positive memories.

Because each day is important, we need to spend those 24 hours doing things together that will give our loved ones the opportunity to say, "Remember when?"

One of my favorite memories about Mom happened when I was twelve. We were at the library where we visited weekly and checked out stacks of books. Each of us – Mom, my sister, my brother and me – were all avid readers. So the weekly trip to the library was a highlight of life, especially in the tumultuous 1960's.

What better way to escape what was happening in our world than to immerse oneself in a fascinating novel or an informative biography. All of us had our favorites and all of us stretched those favorites into other genres – anything to keep reading, to continue learning.

That day, I browsed through the young adult section but could no longer find any books I had not already read. The children's section was boring, my little brother standing before a shelf looking for a chapter book. My sister already engrossed in the latest horse book.

So I wandered into the adult section and chose two books I thought looked interesting. However, when I tried to check them out, the librarian told me, "You are not allowed to check anything out of the adult section."

Mom found me crying behind one of the shelves.

"What's wrong with you?" she asked. Mom was never a nurturer. If anybody cried, there had better be a darned good reason for those salty tears.

I told her what had happened. She grabbed my hand and marched with me to the main desk where she confronted the librarian. "I understand you won't let my daughter check out these books."

"Sh-h-h," said the librarian. "Ma'am, these books are from the adult section and your daughter isn't yet an adult. We cannot allow her to check them out."

Mom stretched into every bit of her 5'8" stature and said, "May I remind you that my taxes pay for the electricity in this building...and the books...and your salary."

"But ma'am," said the librarian in her whispery voice. "We just can't allow...."

"Do I need to speak to your superior or to one of the board members for this public library so my tax money will be used properly? There's nothing in these books that will hurt my daughter, and if she wants to check them out – then she's going to check them out."

"Well, uh, ma'am...." The librarian conferred with another worker, both of them adept at the librarian whisper. Then she returned to my mother who seemed to stand ten feet above me, her arms crossed and a determined look on her face.

"This time," the librarian said, "we'll make an exception."

I left that day with "The Grapes of Wrath" and "The Autobiography of Eleanor Roosevelt." I read them both within a week and loved them. Never again did I have any trouble checking books out of the library.

Somewhere in the library system of my home town, I imagine there still exists a 3x5 card with my name on it and a notation beside it, "Beware of Mother."

Mom may not have been a nurturer, but she fought fiercely for her kids. She taught us to love books, and I treasure the memory of her bold love.

I only wish she could comprehend that I am now a published author. I'll bet if she could see my books on the library shelf, her heart would sing. She would rejoice for all those weeks when she took us to the library.

Another positive memory revolves around Mom's frugal practice of saving money.

As a freshman in high school, I was strongly affected by my peer group. At fourteen, I wanted to fit in and noticed the appearance of other girls in my high school – especially the popular ones.

Bullied in junior high because I wore glasses, I decided I might fit in better with the popular crowd if I could have new frames.

But our family believed in conservative values, saving as much money as possible, and Mom was the queen of saving for a rainy day. We didn't buy anything until we really needed it – and even then – we thought long and hard about it. If we truly needed something, we made it from the tools or ingredients we already owned. Or we used coupons, shopped for the best deals and then

– thought about it again.

When it came to anything as frivolous as new glasses frames, I knew Mom was going to be a hard sell. But surely she would understand my need to fit in with the other girls at school.

I begged, "All the kids have these cool frames. My glasses aren't popular anymore. Don't you think it's time for me to get some new ones? Please!"

Mom peered at me through her own glasses which were probably at least ten years old and definitely out of style. "You don't need different frames, just because the other kids are getting them. We don't buy frames until you need new lenses, and your eyes are just fine."

But teenagers don't give up easily. I brought up the subject every day for at least a week, reporting on the girls in my classes who wore the newest frames. "They look so cool. Everybody talks about my ugly glasses."

Mom must have grown tired of my complaints, because she decided to "make" me some new frames. The creative side of her personality suddenly exploded. "I've decided what we're going to do. These will be the best glasses in the whole school, because they're so different."

I think Mom forgot teenagers don't want to look different. We want to fit in which was the whole point behind my asking for new frames.

To give my new "look" some texture, Mom used a handful of rice kernels and glued them to my glasses frames. Then, to make them even more unique and noticeable, she painted the rice with red fingernail polish.

How mortified I was, an insecure little freshman, as I wore my red rice glasses to school the next day. I struggled through class after class, lunch time and ball games where the entire campus seemed to be laughing at me.

After weeks listening to the snickers of my friends and foes alike, I stopped wearing my glasses. Then I suffered with horrendous headaches and my grades started to suffer.

I complained often. "My eyes hurt, Mom. I have another headache."

She finally decided to take me to the optometrist – just in case – where he pronounced me ready for new lenses as well as new frames. When I returned to school with my brand new glasses, I was overjoyed.

The red rice glasses are now a funny memory, a reminder of who Mom was and how she saved money all those years ago. Only later did I realize she saved so all three of us could attend college without any student loans. She saved to help keep us in decent clothes and now – she lives in a beautiful assisted living facility because she consistently ignored her own needs and saved money for the unknown future.

Alzheimer's cannot steal those memories away nor delete the love and the wisdom behind them. Finding the positive memories buried deep will help us endure the difficult care-giving days.

We owe it to our loved ones to remember – and be grateful.

SUNDOWN HOPE

We first noticed this phenomenon with Dad. During the final stages of his dementia, dusk triggered an inward call. He rose from his chair and began to pace up and down the living room, going nowhere yet constantly moving.

His eyes shone with an almost maniacal light, as if he obeyed a calling we could not see. By that time, he no longer spoke, so we couldn't ask what he was looking for or where he wanted to go. It became his nightly ritual until he could no longer walk. Then we almost wished he could return to the sundown pacing.

Because sundown created some anxiety, I fully expected him to pass away during the dusky hours, when the golden Oklahoma sun begins its descent into the horizon.

But no, he graduated to heaven in the middle of a spring day. His earthly breath simply ceased as he walked away with Jesus.

When Mom worked as a nurse in the hospital, she told me how important it was to work the night shift and watch out for her patients. "If they're going to die," she said, "they'll die at night."

Something about the night conjured up the dark fear of death – all those spooky movies with a full moon shadowing gargantuan monsters. But her beloved did not leave at night, so her theory proved wrong.

But then, the scenario is different when Alzheimer's or dementia capture the brain.

Mom's sundown hours have changed as well. She eats supper early, around 4:30. Perhaps the cooks schedule it early for a purpose, because they know what is coming for many of their residents.

Shortly after supper, Mom moves into her most confused state of the day. She does not pace like Dad, but she is easily distracted and frustrated.

We know better than to visit her in the evening, because she will be concerned about the farm and what is happening there, even though she has not lived in the country for many years. "Who's running the farm now? Is the harvest done? Why am I here?"

In the evenings, she will forget Dad has passed. She will talk about him as if he will come into the room and she must prepare his clothes for the next day.

At dusk, Mom will argue about nonsensical things – what day it is, what year it is, whether we have already celebrated Christmas and whose name she drew and what present she bought.

It doesn't matter what we say or how we try to explain, the shutters of understanding have closed for the day. She is lost within the sunset hours.

An old hymn reminds me of the timelessness of heaven and how sundowner's symptoms will someday cease.

"Beyond the sunset, oh blissful morning
When with our savior, heaven is begun.
Earth's toiling ended, oh glorious dawning
Beyond the sunset, when day is done."

Perhaps hope thrives at sundown, when believers are most restless for heaven, searching for the Savior and for their loved ones who graduated before them. Maybe the elderly saints know each sundown is one day closer to an eternal reunion.

Next time I see Mom at dusk, I will take her hand to calm her and say, "It's okay, Mom. Only a few more sunsets until your journey is over. Be still. The best is yet to be."

FAMILY TIES

Alzheimer's cannot destroy our family ties.

Dad was an introvert while Mom was the talker. Even when dementia destroyed Dad's ability to communicate, Mom kept talking to him. "He can still hear me," she said. "I just wish he could tell me how he feels, tell me anything, talk to me."

Sometimes after supper, she would sit on his lap while they shared a cup of coffee. Their lifelong love commitment remained secure—something not even a memory blip could destroy. They made a great team for fifty-five years and Mom grieved daily as Dad gradually disappeared into the shadows.

Even though Mom's extrovert personality stays intact these days, she seems a bit more closed off since her beloved Hank graduated to heaven. No one but Dad could elicit the same responses from Mom. They knew each other from the quirks in their personalities to the deepest crevices of their souls.

Yet … our family remains strong and devoted to one another. Mom is still and always will be the matriarch who presides over meals. Memories of her strong presence still reverberate around the table as we eat together.

She comes from a long line of pioneer women who raised their children with leather belts or switches from cottonwood trees. Women who knew how to kill a chicken, then strip its feathers and fry it to a golden brown.

Women who worked a job outside the home yet somehow

managed to place a huge meal on the table so the hungry harvest crew found sustenance. Then these resilient women woke early the next morning and did it all over again.

Women who fiercely protected their children, used every resource available and saved enough money so their kids could attend college without fearing debt.

Women who reminded their men to put on a fresh shirt before going to town – even to the local John Deere to pick up a part for the combine.

Women who learned how to manage their own perms and cut the hair of everyone in the family. This is why all my childhood pictures show me grimacing under crooked bangs.

I remember my long line of matriarchs during holiday seasons when I crave my great grandmother's fried green beans and my grandmother's orange Jello salad. I remember Mom's peppernuts every Christmas and wish I wasn't too busy to make them. Her recipe still hides in my recipe box; a maple syrup stain darkens one corner.

During the holidays, we will drive Mom to the same farm where she raised us. I will buy a pecan pie and Cool Whip so she can have her favorite Thanksgiving treat. Somehow, none of us ever learned how to make a really luscious pecan pie. That recipe did NOT travel through our genes.

Mom will sit at the table and occasionally speak. When she does, we will listen – even if it doesn't quite make sense. Because she is the Mom, the grandmother of four and now – great-grandmother of two. She has earned the right to be listened to, to be respected, to be loved.

Later, as she sits in the recliner beside the fire, I will catch her with a look on her face and wonder, *What is she thinking?*

Is she homesick for heaven? Probably. Is she missing her husband, her mother, her grandmothers who taught her so much? Certainly.

Is she remembering those days when she fixed the entire Thanksgiving meal, then organized the clean-up crew, saved all the leftovers and planned how she would make the budget stretch so every child had a special gift at Christmas? I would bet so.

And sometimes – in the glow from the fire – I see in her the features of all the matriarchs before her and I feel gratitude again for the history – the legacy I share of strong women who accomplished so much yet never dwelt on their achievements.

That same strength has been shared with my siblings and I. We have attempted to pass it on to our children so faith, determination and perseverance never diminish throughout our generations.

In the Mennonite church, we used to sing, *"Blessed be the tie that binds, our hearts in Christian love."* As I observe my mother throughout these waning years of her life, those family ties keep us bound together.

This brutal Alzheimer's Disease can never destroy those ties.

LIFELONG HABITS

Alzheimer's Disease cannot change the lifelong habits we practice through the years.

Although some routines will inevitably change as the disease progresses, many of the lifelong habits remain ingrained in the behavior of Alzheimer's patients.

Mom has always loved to read. She goes to the Hospice sales and buys a stack of books. Then she reads the book on the top of the stack. She no longer comprehends what she reads, and she forgets that she read the top book on the stack – so she reads it again. And again. Then she takes the entire stack to another Hospice sale and buys another bunch of books so she can read the top book on the stack.

She is content as she reads because that has always been one of her habits. A stack of books beside her chair is as important as the chocolate cake on her tray at lunch.

She also reads her Bible every day and a page from her "Our Daily Bread" devotional book. This has always been her morning exercise, so even though comprehension is gone, she continues her devotional practice. The Bible remains open all day to that particular passage as if the ghost of her past may sneak a peek and find some comfort in the traditional words.

On Sundays, Mom dresses up for church and carries her Bible with her. Her scarf must be in her pocket in case the Oklahoma wind threatens to mess up her hair. And since Oklahoma ALWAYS has wind whipping through the plains, the scarf completes every outfit. Every Sunday, no matter what, her Bible is with her and her scarf in her pocket. Because that is what she has always done.

She begins every morning with coffee, a little cream, no sugar. Morning coffee has always signaled the beginning of her day. Never tea. Never hot chocolate. Always coffee. Alzheimer's has not yet destroyed her taste buds.

Once I tried to introduce her to Starbucks, but it was too sweet – too strange. "Just Folgers," she said to the perplexed barrista.

Even though osteoporosis has shorted her 5'8" frame, Mom continues to demonstrate careful posture. She walks tall, her congestive heart failure causing a bit of breathlessness – but still – her shoulders back, her head erect, her poise intact.

A cartoon bubble over her head might read, "Don't mess with me. I know who I am."

Like many in her generation, desserts were always part of the meal, so Mom continues to love her sweets. She plays Bingo every week and often wins. With choices of candy, peanuts or trail mix – she always chooses a Snickers bar.

She cannot understand when I turn down cookies or a piece of cake on the menu at the assisted living dining hall. I am gluten free, a concept completely foreign to the wife of a wheat farmer. She tries to cut a piece off her pie for me to, "Taste just a little. You'll like it."

Of course, I will like it, but my body won't. Sometimes, to treat Mom and to apologize for my refusal to taste her dessert, I drive her to Braums for an ice cream cone.

Ice cream has always been the savior of any chaos in life. After the dentist appointment when the filling still tasted metal fresh, Mom took us out for ice cream. After the piano recital, even if we had refreshments at the reception, we still drove to the Tastee Freeze for ice cream.

Maybe because she has been a lifelong reader, Mom hates the television. She calls it, "The Idiot Box" and only watches the news or turns it on for some noise to break the loneliness. Although it was her generation that introduced television to the masses, she never liked it. She would rather sit in her recliner with a book or jump up to take a pie out of the oven – then top it with ice cream.

These habits of life define my mother. They make her authentic and vulnerable yet showcase her personality. They cement our memories of Mom and remind us Alzheimer's cannot steal all of who she is.

The reader, the tall woman, the lover of sweets and hater of TV – these traits characterize my mother and help us cache the remembrance of her life's journey.

Alzheimer's cannot steal her character away.

THE STRENGTH OF FAITH

Alzheimer's cannot destroy faith.

While visiting Mom at the assisted living facility, we decided to go to "church." A pastor would present a brief service and offer encouragement – making Sunday a special day at the "home."

Although Mom was in Stage Five of Alzheimer's, that sacred place within her where God resides had not been forgotten. So she dressed up, picked up her Bible and we walked down the hall toward the dining room.

The room was filled with Alzheimer's and dementia residents in various stages of the disease – beautiful shades of white and gray hair, curly perms and a few shining bald heads of the rare men in the crowd.

I wondered how many residents would gain anything from the service, but I watched as they sang some of their favorite hymns, their faces aglow with the memory of other places – decades past when they sang with their families sitting next to them in wooden pews.

"What a Friend We Have in Jesus."

"Amazing Grace."

"When We All Get to Heaven."

Some of these songs would be included in the programs when these saints graduated to heaven and their families planned memorial services.

Most of the residents hummed along, some fell asleep, a few still knew some of the words. I sang lustily, my mezzo soprano blending with the bass of the pastor. My mother remembered some of the lyrics and hummed through the rest.

Then the pastor said, "Please join me as we all recite Psalm 23."

I suppressed a snicker and thought, *You must be kidding, buddy. These people can't recite a passage of Scripture. They can barely remember their names. No way can they recite an entire Psalm. Alzheimer's is, after all, the memory thief.*

But they surprised me. How deep is that sacred place that resides within the soul! The word of God digs in so intensely – not even a brain disease can disrupt it.

I watched and listened as these dear souls – every single resident in the room – recited word for word the precious Shepherd's Psalm.

"The Lord is my shepherd, I shall not want. He maketh me to lie down in green pastures."

They quoted the King James version, the one they knew best and had memorized years before. None of them missed a beat.

"He leadeth me beside the still waters. He restoreth my soul."

How many of them prayed that God would restore their lives, do a miracle in their bodies and release them from this disease, this long and tragic goodbye?

"He leadeth me in the paths of righteousness for his name's sake."

A righteous life includes reading the word of God and hiding those words in their hearts so that when the end of life comes, when those final years flip over onto the calendar, these residents would hang on to what really matters.

"Yea, though I walk through the valley of the shadow of death, I will fear no evil."

These saints understood the verse because they lived within that valley. I recognized the truth in their eyes, in the faces accessorized with wisdom-carrying wrinkles. They knew this valley and what it foreshadowed yet they recited the verse with joy. They knew only God could help them walk through the last valley unafraid. He would comfort them along the way and never leave them to face it alone.

"Thou preparest a table before me in the presence of mine enemies; thou anointest my head with oil; my cup runneth over."

Food no longer provided comfort because the appetite was gone. The taste buds had forgotten a favorite flavor or the joy of family meals. Yet smiles surfaced around the group – maybe a dim remembrance of God's anointing on a life, the cup of joy that once ran over and now waited its fulfillment.

"Surely goodness and mercy shall follow me all the days of my life...."

My mother, her voice clear, her eyes bright – solid in her faith and waiting for her timeline to end.

"And I shall dwell in the house of the Lord forever."

I could not speak. Tears choked me as I acknowledge that divine place deep within us, the sanctuary of the soul that cannot be stolen by whatever is happening in the brain.

Alzheimer's cannot and will never destroy faith.

Amen and amen.

THE JOURNEY CONTINUES

As of this writing – as 2017 begins – my mother's brave heart still beats.

She has merged into the sixth stage of Alzheimer's where life resonates increasingly in a confusing pattern. Although she seems to remember her family members, she has memory lapses that cause fear and concern. Yet she has learned to cope throughout this journey, a living example of how the brain functions – even beyond disease.

We aren't sure when Mom says, "Hi, kiddo" who she's really remembering in her plaque-infested brain. But we internalize the greeting, hoping she still remembers who we are and our connection as family members.

Many of her routines continue as she still dresses herself. But she has lost several items of clothing and we are perplexed as to whether doctor and dentist appointments are still necessary. At what point does a caregiver exclaim, "Enough!"

Mom has lost some of her teeth. A hole gaps in her smile. The dentist cemented a bridge into her mouth, but she dug it out. The physical strength of a demented mind defies logic.

Relationships no longer make logical sense as she has forgotten her best friend still lives while the spouse is now gone. She reverses who is married to whom, who is alive and who lies beneath the Mennonite cemetery soil. Conversations about the dead and the living merge into one matrix of confusion. Yet the fact that she can still speak is a blessing.

Ironically, her physical body is in good shape. She walks upright and unlike many residents in assisted living, she doesn't need a walker or a cane. At 89 years of age, Mom acts spry. Perhaps all the years of exercise, working on the farm and carrying herself with perfect posture have transitioned into healthy bones, strong joints and functioning organs.

It is her brain that continues to limp, skipping a beat now and then, mixing up words and responding to life with a combination of paranoia and anger.

I wonder when the phone call will come, and I pray every day God will allow her to slip painlessly into eternity – before she has to move into Memory Care – before she becomes bedridden and completely out of her mind. She would so hate that.

I hope God will appear to her one day, hold out his hand and say, "Come home." That she will run toward the Light and be reunited with her beloved Hank.

The human body is a perplexing albeit amazing machine and often it is harder to die than it is to live. But each of us has a timeline – my mother included – and someday she will reach the end of her journey.

In the meantime, we continue to care for her, to pray over her and beg God that whatever gene caused this memory thief will not be passed down to her children and grandchildren.

However long God grants her, we know she lived her life well, graduated to heaven and received her reward beyond the clouds.

I love you forever, Mom. I miss the woman you once were, but I know this disease occurs only for a season and seasons always end.

See you in the great beyond – when your memory will be clear and every cell alive with the glory of a pure eternity.

I look forward to that day.

ABOUT THE AUTHOR

RJ Thesman has been a writer since she flipped open her Red Chief tablet and scribbled her first story. She is the author of The Reverend G trilogy, published by CrossRiver Media – the story of a woman minister and her journey through Alzheimer's Disease:

"The Unraveling of Reverend G"
"Intermission for Reverend G"
"Final Grace for Reverend G"

Thesman has a BS in Education and is a certified life coach, a writing coach and a Stephen Minister. She has published over 700 articles and her work has appeared in 14 anthologies.

She is a professional member of the American Association of Christian Counselors, the National Association of Professional Women, the Kansas Authors Club, the Heart of America Christian Writer's Network and the Fellowship of Christian Writers.

Thesman enjoys teaching workshops, speaking at various venues, reading, gardening and cooking – especially anything with blueberries.

You can follow RJ Thesman on Facebook, Twitter, LinkedIn and Goodreads. Check out her website: RJThesman.net